Level Par

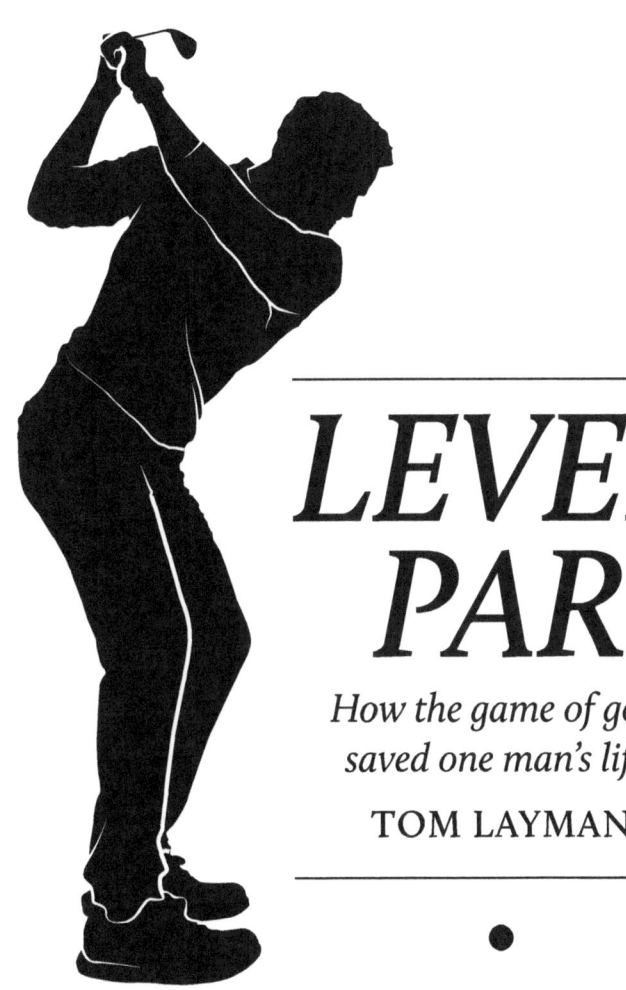

LEVEL
PAR

*How the game of golf
saved one man's life.*

TOM LAYMAN

Briley & Baxter Publications | Plymouth, Massachusetts

ISBN: 978-1-961978-67-6

Book Design: Amy Deyerle-Smith

"Golf is the closest game to the game we call life. You get bad breaks from good shots; you get good breaks from bad shots - but you have to play the ball where it lies."

- Bobby Jones

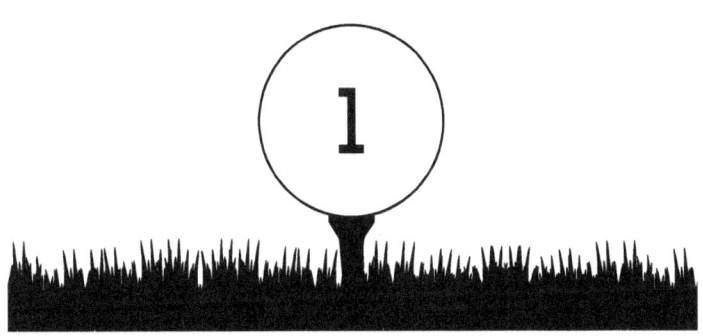

Jonesy was very quiet. It wasn't like him. Ever since he spent time on his deathbed battling a nasty fungal infection, he seemingly always had something to say. Maybe it was the near-death experience a year ago that gave him the extra motivation to let his thoughts out.

His message is always something positive these days. The old cliché "take every day as a blessing" comes to mind. (Again, a result of almost dying, I'm guessing.) I never really believed in it all— at least I didn't until I got serious about life and started taking accountability for my part in it.

Nevertheless, my best friend of more than twenty years and his silence were suddenly very apparent and out of character. Had he been like this all day, and I just hadn't noticed? Come to think of it, the last couple of hours were kind of a blur.

I watched as he stared straight ahead, peering from under the brim of his black hat pulled down just above his eyebrows. Sweat stains formed around his temples from carrying my golf bag on an unusually soupy, New England day in the middle of May. Jonesy's focus was lasered in, straight ahead. He clutched his yardage book firmly in his right hand, holding it near his face, deep in thought. One glance at it. One glance up. He continued this pattern for what felt like eterni-

1

ty, until he finally looked in my direction.

"Okay, bud, take it up the left-hand side and put a good swing on it. Let's bring this thing home," he said while holding my gaze for the first time since I became aware of his odd behavior.

"Bring this home?" What did he mean by that? Off in the distance was the par-four, 460-yard, eighteenth hole at Crestview Country Club. The hole begged you to hit your tee shot into the welcoming pond on the right-hand side just off the fairway. Just my luck, as I have always had a natural left-to-right fade with my driver. Jonesy knew that maybe better than anyone. It was a shot I probably rehearsed a million times in my lifetime, so it shouldn't be an issue.

But it was what Jonesy said that perplexed me.

"Bring this home." Those words stuck out to me. He said it with such intensity and with purpose that it made me stop right there on the tee box.

I looked around and started to take notice of my surroundings. About twenty to thirty people had gathered around my group on the eighteenth tee. I scanned the crowd quickly and didn't recognize a single person. During U.S. Open Qualifying, it's not out of the ordinary to have a few onlookers, like friends, family, and other players, come to see how the other competitors were doing.

This felt different.

I had never seen this many people watch me play before in my life, and they all had this same nervous energy as if they were about to witness something.

My heart started beating a touch faster. My palms began to sweat. A tightness around my neck and throat intensified with each passing second. At that moment, I realized something was happening on the course.

These strangers were here to see me.

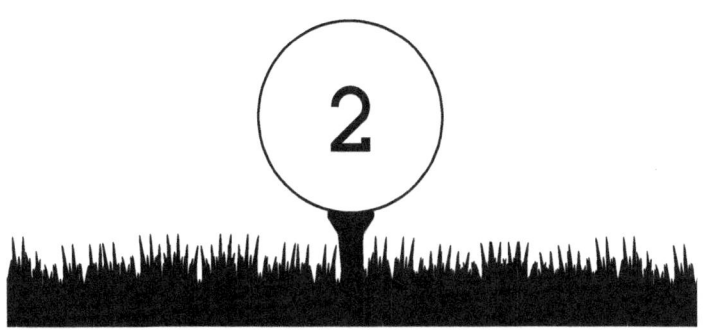

The United States Golf Association holds qualifying tournaments for golfers each year to see if they can play their way into one of the biggest and most grueling tests of golf in this country—The U.S. Open Championship.

The field is open to anybody who fits the criteria for qualifying. Basically you have to be really good at golf just to play in a local qualifying tournament to make it one more step to "Golf's Longest Day": a thirty-six hole grind for a handful of spots to play in the U.S. Open.

The fields usually consist of former professionals who are still hanging on to the dream, stud college players at some of the most prestigious golf programs in the country, and local legends who think they have what it takes for a few rounds with the big boys.

You could say I had a category of my own: Former junior golfer who ruined himself with drugs and alcohol after dipping a pinky toe into the mini-tour world in Florida more than a decade ago. Sure, I could play, and at one point, I thought I was destined for something else. There certainly weren't any kids at this tournament asking for the autograph of Jake Steadman. Some probably thought I shouldn't even be there at all by looking at me, and I wouldn't blame them.

I'm not a junior golfer anymore. I'm thirty-six, certainly not overpowering anyone with my five-foot, ten-inch frame, and a belly that overhangs my belt strap. I'm not striking fear into the hearts of my competition. Am I the worst-looking specimen in the group? No. But yet, here I am, way past my prime, trying to prove to everyone that I have what it takes to earn my spot.

For all of my current physical limitations, the one thing I still have is a great golf swing. From the time I came out of the womb, my old man placed a club in my hand and marked me destined for greatness. The problem is that the game is called "golf," and not "golf swing," and the mental fortitude and intangibles that are needed to be considered one of the best golfers weren't imparted to me, despite my father's forecasting for great things.

The magnitude of where I am hits me like a ton of bricks. You know those moments when an athlete comes out of the "zone" and the walls come caving in? That was me. The impostor syndrome and being found out landed right in my lap, because my journey to this spot was littered with what-could-have-beens and wasted talent and a potential waste of life until just over a year before.

Depending on the size of the field, there are usually only one or two spots allotted to the top finishers in the local qualifying sectionals, and the words "bring it home" from Jonesy made me realize that I was four shots away from living out the dream of so many. Suddenly, it became hard to fathom that I, Jake Steadman, could be one step closer to teeing it up with Tiger Woods and all the other great golfers in the game when, just thirteen months ago, I was contemplating ending it all.

My thoughts went into overdrive. A cold feeling crept over my bones, and my mouth went incredibly dry. I backed away and didn't start my normal routine. It was like my body had no idea what to do. Being anywhere else sounded like the best option for me at this moment.

Jonesy must have noticed that whatever zone I was in was now gone.

When he looked in my direction, he had that look, like it was his fault for breaking my concentration. The cardinal rule of a caddie is to never put a negative thought in your player's head before they are ready to play. His method wasn't wrong; I was just way over my head, and now I knew it.

"Jakey. Look at me, bro," Jonesy said sternly, drawing my attention and holding my gaze. "What you've done over these last seventeen holes has been nothing short of amazing. These guys haven't been through half the shit you have in your life. They haven't been through half the shit we've been through together the last year. All of this you earned. All the bullshit you've put yourself through. All that has happened has put you here. Right here, right now."

The tidal wave of racing thoughts running through my head started to subside a bit as Jonesy kept talking.

"All you need is four shots. Four seconds of greatness and we've got it. Now aim to the left side of the fairway and let it rip like you've been doing all day. I'm proud of you and I trust you."

Trust was something I didn't have from anyone, not even myself. My driver felt like a lead pipe in my hand. The crowd felt like a gallery five rows deep at Augusta National. But Jonesy was right. I was nobody before, and would most likely be nobody, no matter how this thing shook out to the people watching.

This was my opportunity to earn something for the first time in my life, to know that I followed through and put in the work for myself, not for anyone else.

I needed the equivalent of four seconds of greatness like Jonesy said. That fraction of a moment when the clubhead meets the ball. But first, I needed the pumping in my chest and the tightness in my throat to allow me to take a breath without feeling like death was coming next.

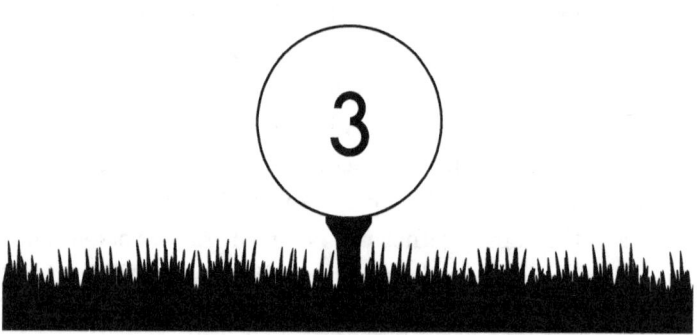

3

Golf is a game of precision, accuracy, timing, and patience. Patience was never my thing. It's not that I didn't possess patience; it just wasn't passed down the Steadman family tree.

Jack "Jackie" Steadman is my father, and his life has always consisted of a combination of self-destruction, anger, the occasional happiness, and a stiff bourbon. His mood depends on the day or the scenario, or even what may happen to him at that very moment. He loves golf. He loves booze. He loves women. Most importantly, he has always loved how people revered his son with the golden golf swing.

I got into the game of golf in diapers, and I didn't have much of a choice. Jackie wouldn't have had it any other way. When the Masters came on every April, Jackie would remind me that one day I would make the family proud and wear one of the green jackets they put on the winners in Butler Cabin. He would usually pass out shortly after the tournament, right there on the edge of his chair, and getting a grown man to bed as a young child was no easy feat.

When I was a kid, it was clear that golf made Jackie happy, and as his only child, I wanted to make him happy. The alternative was not something that was fun to deal with.

My father wasn't wrong about my natural talent for playing golf. The swing came easily to me as a three-year-old. My childhood was spent at Jackie's home golf course, Ridgeway Country Club. It was no secret that Jackie was entrenched as one of the main characters at the club, always sitting in his favorite seat on the patio with a cigar in his hand, staring out towards the green, waiting for his boy to come up the final hole. He would tell a tall tale about his most recent round or my feats as a golfer. His cackle would bellow down the fairway every time I walked towards the clubhouse. It was like the soundtrack of my childhood. I almost perfectly memorized the stories he'd unknowingly repeat because he would get so plastered, he would forget who and what he told to the gallery that was there to see him. (At least he thought they were there to see him.)

Jackie made sure I was always there whenever he was, which was most days after school and for hours on end through the weekends. I didn't play organized sports or really make all that many friends outside the boundaries of Ridgeway. It was where Jackie wanted to be, and I had no say in the matter.

I liked it, though. When Jackie was playing, I was practicing my chipping and putting. When he was drinking, I was on the course after all the members finished their morning rounds, and the afternoon tee sheet was light. From sunup to sundown, I learned the game by myself. My game matured, just as Jackie predicted, as a young junior golfer on the circuit at Ridgeway. It was a small group of golfers, but the competition was pretty good. It's where I met Jonesy for the first time. We were just a couple of young kids, but he and I had a bond because our situations were somewhat similar. Both his old man and mine felt that golf greatness was in our futures. But the way the two men went about promoting the avenue to get to those goals was completely different. Jonesy had a regular family and excelled in other sports. I had Ridgeway and Jackie, and there was no off switch there.

Proving that I was good at something fueled me in those early days. I won most of the junior tournaments at the club. I cleaned up in the drive, chip, and putt every single year until I was about twelve years old. I spent way more time at the club than these other kids out of sheer inability to do anything else. Some of the best prep schools started to take notice of my golf prowess and would show up to watch me hit balls and play.

Most of the coaches would meet Jackie and leave unimpressed. Not if you asked him. But they saw something of a red flag in the way that Jackie was managing me, and, even more so, himself. No matter what they thought, golf was coming easily for me, and me closing out matches and tournaments was becoming almost customary at Ridgeway. There were no failures in those early years, and the ego I developed around Ridgeway started to reach a level that shouldn't have been earned by any twelve-year-old kid.

"You good?" I heard Jonesy say, not realizing that I had completely zoned out during my warmup routine on the tee box. The driver was still swinging back and forth in my right hand as I looked ahead. My brain is not where it should be at this moment. This is exactly what started happening to me in my teens. Out of nowhere, my brain would warp into another dimension, and my golf game suffered. It was like I couldn't keep track of my thoughts. Every moment of my life would come up in a flash. Every mistake. Every cringey memory. Every disappointment that I felt from my dad in those painful car rides home. It was happening again in this crucial moment of the round.

"Yeah...yeah. I'm good, Jonesy," I said, fully knowing I was not. "Keep it up the left side and stay down and through it just like we talked about," I reassured him, knowing that nothing was assuring about the way I felt. The mind is something that must be controlled to play great golf, even if just for a second. I was failing miserably at controlling anything.

At some point I'd have to hit this thing and accept my fate. I took a giant breath and approached the ball.

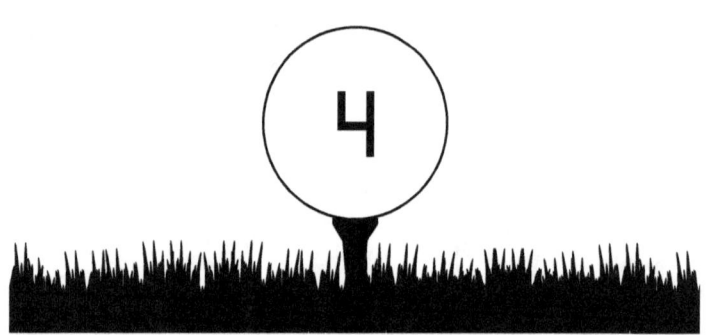

I had one memory playing in my head as I fixed my attention on my target.

"There is nothing wrong with your golf swing," Tom Clark said matter-of-factly. He then placed the butt end of his club against my forehead. "It's what's in here that is your problem."

Tom's lessons over the last eight months flooded into my memory bank right there over my tee shot, causing a lot of mental noise. There's no one way to hit a golf ball, but there are a lot of wrong ways to do it. Filling yourself with swing thoughts while on the golf course is probably the one thing you do not want to do before the biggest drive of your life. Tom taught hundreds, if not thousands, of golfers during his fifty years as a PGA professional. Some went on to better their handicaps, and a few went on to good careers as professional golfers across the world. The man knew what he was talking about. So, I was lucky to connect with him in some ways that I still don't understand.

"It's who you are and what you do," he would say repeatedly. But there was one caveat in his delivery and message... he knew that people could change.

I hoped he was right.

The eighteenth hole at Crestview was trouble for my driver swing with water on the right-hand side. Jonesy alluded to it. I knew it. I also had no idea how I was swinging earlier because all of that happened in a flow state, and now the only things flowing were the thoughts of everything that had ever gone wrong in my life, right between my ears.

My driver has always had a natural fade to it, even when I hit it on the screws. I like to call it a "baby fade." It's my tried-and-true shot that has been a very good friend off the tee. But the stakes for the thousands of other times I've hit weren't nearly as high as they were right now.

My fatal "miss", and there have been plenty of those, is to get a little too quick and extend early, either sending the ball a mile left by flipping my hands over or a mile right by holding on and not letting go of the club. In this case, left wouldn't kill me. Right would be death.

The end of the clubhouse was the direct line that I was looking at. There was a flagpole just off the left side of the green, way off in the distance, that was a perfect line to start my fade. I set my club and then set my body parallel to my line. All of these steps sound so prescriptive, but when you are a self-taught golfer and then actually get true professional direction, you start to run through the checklist like a surgeon does before a major procedure.

This wasn't brain surgery or life and death. But it was close in golfing terms.

My left arm felt tight as I tried to waggle some nervous energy out of my system. My grip was stronger than usual. Loose grip pressure and swinging free have always been a great recipe for me. I was going to have to close this thing out a different way. I took one last breath and started to move the club back away from the ball. In a flash, the driver and ball met for what I hoped was my first second of greatness.

I could tell we were safe as soon as the ball started its flight, even if I didn't get all of it. It soared a little left of the flagpole as I caught it ever so slightly off the heel. Jonesy was leaning to his left, trying to help guide the ball. I knew we were alright. Not great. But alright. It wasn't my usual distance off the tee. I was just glad to make contact in this scenario. The ball started curving over the line of the flagpole and landed safely on the right side of the fairway. We were dry. I could hear the crowd murmur as they let out a round of applause, marveled by my calmness under pressure. I picked up my tee, kept my head down, and did my best to ignore the patrons. If they honestly knew what was going on in my head, they wouldn't be clapping.

Jonesy came and grabbed my driver, quickly putting the headcover back on the club. I didn't need that thing anymore. The first job was to get off the tee and give myself a chance. I had done that. The hardest job would be up to me, to keep my brain here in the present moment and focused on the task at hand, instead of thinking about every little thing that happened in my very messy life up until this point.

The longest hole of my life was just beginning.

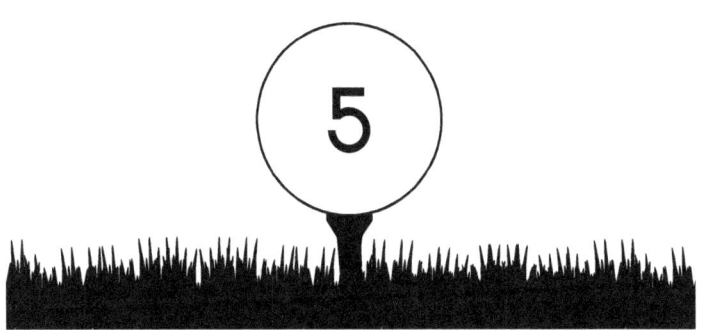

5

"**Y**our whole life, you've been told you had a great golf swing, which you do," Tom said on a rainy Sunday morning from inside his hitting bay at Clark Golf & Practice facility. "But the game is called golf and not golf swing."

It was something that Tom Clark used to say to me nonstop during our lessons. Tom loved the power of repetition when coaching his golfers. Not just in the way he taught the golf swing, but in the way he spoke to you. I think he was just hoping things would stick with his pupils. The best way to do that was to infiltrate your mind with repetition and cold, hard truth.

Tom was not a big man. He stood at five feet seven inches and had a slender frame. His glasses made his eyes appear bigger, and the grey hair on his head was holding strong. At just about seventy years old, he glided back and forth in his rocking chair during lessons and only got to his feet to deliver messages when he was trying to drive a point home.

I always listened just a little more intently when he got out of the chair. Our lessons had turned into the highlights of my week ever since I came back to Massachusetts from Florida a year ago. I started to truly see some changes in my game that had never materialized with years and years of trying to fix something on my own.

The last time I hit balls in Florida, a few years prior, I could feel a panic attack coming on. It was manic. I was sweating, breathing heavily, and was probably three days into a bender that would have stopped a normal person's heart. Having Tom there and being sober now made the sessions more fun. Tom had heard of me as a junior golfer. His style wasn't to extend an invite to potential clients, but he would take you on if you sought him out.

I was no longer the twelve-year-old that he probably could have molded into a polished young golfer. The person hitting golf balls in front of him as he rocked back and forth was very obviously beaten down by life and scarred by the lofty expectations that were not met. The toll of years of hard living had done a number on my outsides. I was working on it but comfortable in my skin, I certainly was not.

I knew I needed Tom if I wanted to find any kind of form to my golf game after years of abuse. I asked him to tear me down and bring me back up. I didn't care how long it took, but I wanted to play good golf again, even if it was just for me. I wanted Tom to treat me like a student who had never picked up a club in my life. Quite frankly, I was that, in a way. My handicap still said "1.4" in the official golf ranking system, but numbers sometimes don't tell the whole story.

He wouldn't take a dime from me for any lesson, which I found odd. It never made sense why one of the best teachers around would take on a "never was," a true reclamation project, let alone refuse to be compensated for the challenge. His compliments were few and far between. You had to earn them. It was so different from my father, who would heap praise, mostly to make himself feel better, even if my play was worthy of it.

"Good," Tom would say sharply when a task was completed satisfactorily. That's when you know you did something well, when the octave in his voice rose while saying the word "good." "There is no way in hell you will ever go left with that golf swing. Good job."

His teachings were all about eliminating the left side of the golf course. "If you can do that," he would tell me, "You can improve your scores." But eliminating things was a skill that had always been hard for me to do. I had lived with so many bad habits, too much anxiety, terrible nightmares, benders that would turn into months without truly knowing where time had gone.

Tom's lessons weren't just about golf, they were about life, and as I strolled up the fairway, I realized how much further along in life I was from where I had been. I smiled and realized what Tom had been teaching me stuck. But man was it hard.

Jonesy was a few paces ahead of me on our walk towards my ball in the fairway. The crowd had created some distance between myself and my fellow playing members. Jonesy wanted to get a good look at the lie before I got up to my approach shot. He always wanted to be prepared, and he was always looking out for me.

When he turned back in my direction after analyzing our lie, he had a very un-Jonesy-like look to him. I knew something was up.

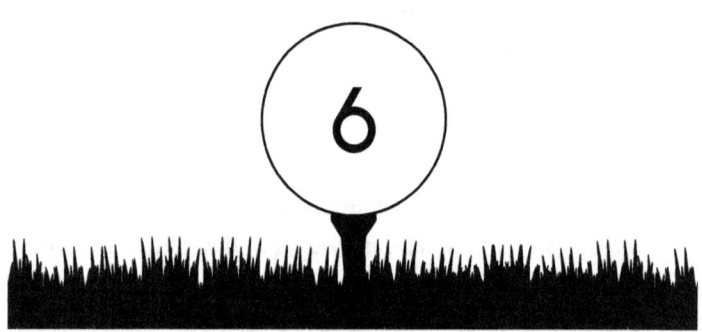

The television was turned up to an ungodly volume. A metallic taste filled my mouth and a pack's worth of smoked cigarette butts filled up a pizza box on the coffee table. My right eye was slightly swollen, and my vision was blurry.

It was Tuesday. Or Wednesday? I wasn't exactly sure. After finally getting my vision to settle like water finding its level, I realized I was in my apartment and, judging by the sky, it was sometime before seven a.m.

I reached for the remote with one arm and knocked over a few beer bottles, trying to grab something that felt like... a pistol? It was. Where did that come from? I was startled a bit when I heard what I thought was my phone vibrate from somewhere in the room. I looked around, confused. I had no idea where that buzzing was coming from.

My place was a sty. There were two bottles of prescription medication tipped over and splayed out all over the place. The remnants of cocaine frosted a broken shard from a mirror. It was like a war zone. I stumbled to my feet and tried to follow the buzzing. My head was wobbly, and I felt a fire in my right nostril. I deciphered that the vibration was coming from somewhere under the absolute disaster of a mess in the kitchen.

Who the fuck was calling me at this time?

I looked at my phone and it was Jonesy's wife. I had never spoken to Bri on the phone before, but I had her number saved from when Jonesy was down to caddy for me years ago. She was not my biggest fan.

I tried to collect myself before answering the phone.

"Hello," I said half awake and sounding like a bag of shit.

"Jake. Jake, can you hear me?" Bri said. I realized I hadn't turned down the volume on the TV yet, and it could be heard straight through the phone. It sounded like I was at a busy bar at seven a.m.

"Yes, yes, hold on," I said, stumbling over to hit the power button on the side of the TV. I was sure Bri could hear the beer bottles and other debris get kicked around.

"What's up, Bri?" I asked, kind of confused as to why she was calling.

"I'm calling because Jonesy's sick and we aren't sure what's going on. You need to figure out a way to get home as soon as possible. He would want you here," she said in a serious tone.

I wasn't sure if I was dreaming or not. I also knew this was not a call Bri wanted to make.

"We're at Mass General. Just...come. Quickly. I've got to go, the doctors are here," she said and hung up the phone.

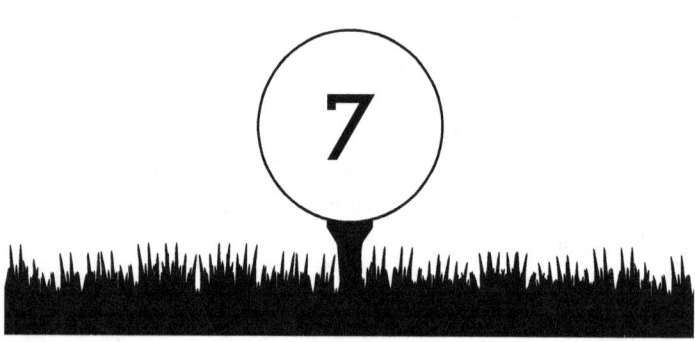

7

Walking up towards Jonesy, who still had this disappointed look on his face, brought me back to a moment at Ridgeway years ago.

"You should have seen the drive Jakey hit on number four. I've never seen anything like it," Jackie said to his captivated audience at Ridgeway.

I could hear my old man's conversation from my table. He was bellied up at the bar while I sat and had my post-round hot dog and Shirley Temple. I was ten years old. Holding court at the nineteenth hole at Ridgeway was Jackie's sermon. It was where he could spread the word about his kid's golf game. Anyone who would catch a sight of me on the course could tell I had a tremendous golf swing from an early age, and nobody at Ridgeway could forget about it because Jackie would brag about how well I was coming along in his eyes.

"I don't even think Beamer could hit it that far," Jackie said in the direction of the longest hitter at the club. Beamer raised his glass, and you could tell there was a smirk that said, "Oh yah, well fuck you too Jackie."

"Always be a member at a club," Jackie would constantly say. "You never know when you are going to need it."

Everything out of his mouth was delivered like a life lesson, especially when his post-round lasted longer than his time on the course. It was ironic because the life lessons came from a guy who desperately needed a lesson in how to live his own life.

He wasn't wrong about my golf game, though. As I got stronger and bigger in my early teens, I got better and better. The better I got, the more embellished the stories grew from Jackie's mouth to God's ear. Some were spot on, while others were just old wives' tales. In twenty years, who knew what those stories would end up sounding like?

There was no doubt where Jackie envisioned my life going. As his only kid, I wanted to make that happen. When you're young, you don't see the faults of your parents. You don't truly understand what adults even are, let alone how they are flawed. You just know that it's your dad, and if this is his dream, then it should be your dream too. Besides, it felt good to be good at something and get the adoration from my dad (and a bunch of older men at the club.) It was driving my ego, even though I was still only playing inside the walls of Ridgeway.

There was a whole other golf world out there where kids were playing against each other in tournaments. Jackie didn't have the time to do that, so he pumped my tires at Ridgeway and said my game would travel everywhere I went. He would "make sure of it" (even though he did nothing to instill a discipline of hard work in my game or life, and those cracks would start to surface pretty quickly after my game started to go downhill.)

As I approached Jonesy, I could hear my old man's cackle coming down the fairway. It didn't make any sense why it was so audible or why I was even hearing it at this moment. I felt like that ten-year-old kid waiting for a hot dog. While Jonesy was ready to deliver me some news, my brain was just getting started to relive every moment where my life started going wrong.

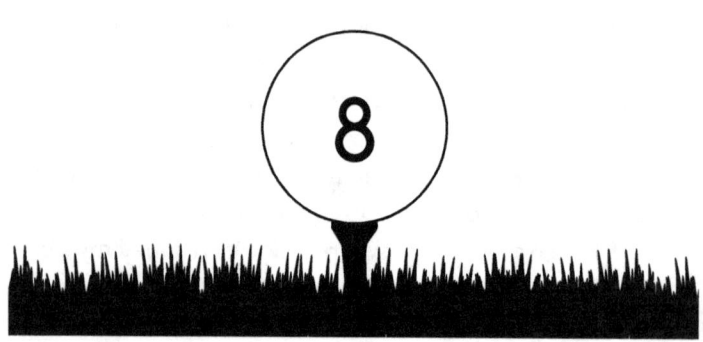

8

When it was time for me to leave the cozy confines of Ridgeway and start competing on a bigger junior circuit to get my name out there, I certainly looked the part. The competition was better once I turned fourteen for sure, but I had the game to compete. I could hit it as far as anyone. My irons were just as good as some of the best players in the state, and my upbringing on the fast greens at Ridgeway made me an above-average putter for my age group.

All the things were coming into place just as Jackie had said they would, except for one thing.

I was having an incredibly hard time closing out tournaments and matches at this level. The wins came easily at Ridgeway, where I knew every nook and cranny of the golf course like the back of my hand. It wasn't the case anywhere else I played. Jonesy, even in my corner back then, would always tell me it was a matter of time before I broke through. I guess he was always optimistic, even as a kid, which drove me nuts.

I didn't share that sentiment deep down. Small cracks in my confidence started to form. There was a deep rage that was bubbling inside of me. It had probably been there for years and years. As I got older, I realized how different my upbringing was from everyone else's. Jonesy and all my peers seemed to have two parents at home, multiple siblings, and even a dog with a white picket fence.

I had my old man and Ridgeway. There was no balance. My whole life was caught up in this game and the expectations that I needed to fulfill. The game of golf, which was a sanctuary to me growing up, was turning into a place of nightmares, especially on the last hole of these bigger tournaments. Nine times out of ten, I would be right there at the end, but a missed putt here, a wayward drive there, a mental mistake or a poorly executed chip, and it was always me watching someone else celebrate a well-earned victory.

Whether it be on the practice range or the putting green, there were never any issues. The competition would watch me hit balls before the round or watch me nail twenty-five-foot putts on the practice green and wonder who I was. When I'd get to crunch time on the course, that aura would evaporate.

Jackie wasn't a happy camper when this happened either. The truth was, we didn't have much money. Jackie was holding on to his membership for dear life after his hours got cut at his job. He was practically grandfathered into Ridgeway, and the Board at the club did what they could to acquiesce to his needs. There wasn't any money left over for lessons or coaches or anything else to take my game to the next level. There were just disappointments and angry questions from my father as to why I was completely folding every single time I got to the course.

I didn't have Tom yet to drop an anecdote or give me a swing tip, so when I failed, I would tinker with my swing. When the ball didn't hit the center of the face, I would head to the range and start playing around with my grip or my stance. Every swing was something different. Consistency was nowhere to be found during my practice sessions. I was still good enough to be in it on natural talent, but where the ball was going to go was a guessing game at times, and there's a huge difference between a tee shot on the first hole and the eighteenth when a match is on the line. The pressure was crumbling me to the point where I knew exactly when the wheels were going to fall off, and they never went back on.

Throwing clubs, swearing, not being a gentleman of the game, as they say in golf. All of it was on full display. Dealing with failure was my biggest flaw. That work needs to be done from within, but I didn't have the patience or the discipline, and letting down my father every time I played golf was breaking me down. At fourteen years old and with an ego built up from a young age, I was not equipped to handle any of it.

My home life was getting rough. Jackie came to very few of the tournaments. When he did make it, he would be liquored up, trying to make small talk with the parents. We all knew what he was doing. He was looking for a new audience for his sermons. His schtick at Ridgeway wasn't translating to these more uptight golf tournaments, and when you brag about the kid who isn't sweeping the leaderboards, your stories of grandeur don't hit as well. His frustrations with that were taken out on me when I didn't perform.

The rides home when he did come see me were some the worst. Instead of building me up, I had to answer for every single mistake I made and why I made it. It was like getting a microphone shoved in your face after missing a putt to win a major championship. Only, the person peppering you with questions was the one person you wanted to go to for comfort and understanding. Tough love was fine. This was something different.

The anxiety was starting to build within me day by day, match by match, hole by hole.

It was only a matter of time until the apple didn't fall far from the tree.

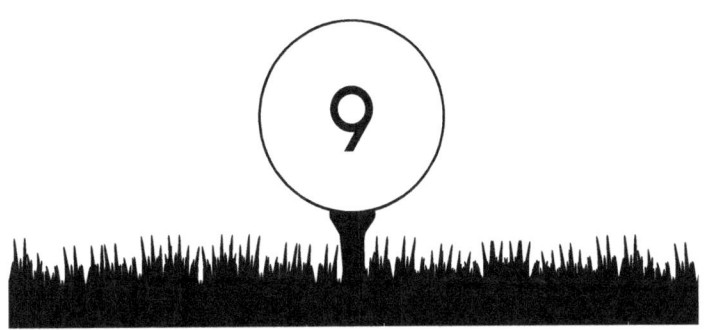

9

There was a loud bang on my door. Then another one. Bang. Bang. Bang.

The next one finally jolted me from the couch. As my heart rate started to come down, I realized I was in my apartment. It looked like a sidewalk in midtown Manhattan.

"Jake, are you in there?" the voice screamed from behind the door. Whoever it was, they didn't seem very happy.

I stumbled to my feet and nearly fell over. I was dizzy, and the fire in my nostrils told me that a bag of cocaine was on the menu last night. Those mornings were always the toughest. I didn't dabble all the time, but put me around the right crew, and I would be the one talking about God knows what at four-thirty a.m. in a random kitchen with people I barely knew. There was nothing positive about those interactions, but what else was there to do when your golf game was floundering and your drive to do anything in life was almost gone?

The voice behind the door was growing more agitated. As I got closer, I realized it was Jonesy. I sprang from the couch, ready to face my shame head-on with my oldest friend.

The last thing I remember is we were at a bar in downtown Tampa, and Jonesy had just met us. He was in town to caddie for me in the biggest tournament of the mini-tour season. I had called him for help a few weeks prior because it was kind of a last lifeline. There was nobody else that I trusted to help me out of this rut that I was digging myself into down here. I thought getting a familiar face on my bag might help me sort out some of the wrongs that had developed in my game.

Bri and Jonesy were pretty serious in their relationship, and they had moved in together. She wasn't a fan of me and didn't like the thought of her potential future husband hanging out with the people I associated with. She thought it was a bad idea for him to come down. She even told him when I was on the phone with him. I heard every word and accepted whatever fate would happen.

Being my oldest and only friend, he told me he would be there. When I opened the door, I could read on his face that he couldn't believe this was the person whom he agreed to help. Here I was, strung out on cocaine and disheveled by every sense of the word. When Jonesy gave me the once over you could tell he was incredibly disappointed.

"Jake, you are so late," he said. The edge in his voice was something he couldn't hide. My shoulders curled up, and I got very small. This was not fun for me either.

I had moved down to Florida shortly after finishing high school. My alcohol addiction started when I turned fifteen and it was peaking pretty hard down here. The sun was always shining. The bars were always open. The women and the parties were always happening. I fit right in.

I hadn't set myself up to do anything with school or really any other career outside of the game of golf. I came down here to caddy and play in some of the mini-tours to earn a little cash. The booze I used to calm my nerves, which had allowed me to play good golf and close out a couple of tournaments, was a full-fledged problem at this point. But I thought I was playing well enough to make a little bit of money, caddy on the side, and keep this thing going for a few more years. Besides, I didn't have any other skills other than what I was doing.

Jonesy knew I was kind of on my last legs down here and thought he might be able to help. I was certain he could when we talked at dinner. He told me Bri wouldn't let him stay at my place, so he grabbed a cheap hotel in town. He knew I was half in the bag at dinner, but didn't say anything about it. I told him all my stories about how I was really doing well and playing okay. The Jackie in me was really laying on thick. I seemed to have gotten the storyteller trait from my pops.

Under this false bravado was a scared shitless kid. I knew I was heading for a final breaking point, and this was my last effort to do something about it. The final thing I remember from Jonesy was him telling me to get home and get some sleep before he went back to his hotel. I vaguely remember agreeing. Based on the shape I was in this morning, I didn't deliver on that promise.

"Bud, are you OK?" he asked. The tone in his voice was more concerned than pissed off at this point.

"I ... I ... I just got to take a shower, and we will be on our way," I said.

"You are on the tee in an hour. It takes us forty-five minutes to get to the course. I've been banging on this door and calling you for the last hour. You got three minutes to get your shit together. I'll get your clubs and everything you need. Just make yourself presentable," he said.

I knew I had fucked up. I darted off to the shower and heard Jonesy rummaging through my shitty apartment, mumbling under his breath. My recipe for the usual hangover of this magnitude was to lie in the shower and fall asleep with it on for an hour or so. Usually, I'd throw up all over myself. At least I was doing it in a place where I could just wash it off my pathetic body.

I threw myself into a cold shower and let out a scream. I didn't have time to wallow in my self-pity. There was half a beer in the shower, and I chugged it in search of my equilibrium.

The car ride was silent. Honestly, there wasn't much to

say. I looked at my phone and realized I got a text right after dinner. There was a free table open at a club in Tampa, and I didn't have to pay anything to get in. There were girls and bottle service and everything I could want. Plus, it was all covered. I just had to pick up some party favors. (Which I must've obliged based on the feeling of an ice pick being hammered into my brain.)

Jonesy finally broke the silence.

"Bud, I'm worried about you. But let's get through this round. We can talk about what needs to happen next once you're done," he said.

Jonesy knew it was going to be a long day on the course. He hadn't seen me swing in a few years and wasn't convinced I was going to be able to make contact with the ball in my current condition. I rummaged through my pockets for a cigarette, and the remnants of the bag of cocaine fell out onto the middle console.

Jonesy looked at it and gripped the wheel a little tighter. There was nothing I could say at that moment. There was no sorry. No apologies. I had to just accept that I was a shitty friend and probably a shittier human. But man, could I swing a golf club.

We arrived at the golf course with about ten minutes to spare. I rushed to the registration, and they let me know that I was on the tee next. I had just enough time to get to the bathroom and down the nip of Jack Daniels that I had found in the pocket of my golf bag. I was grateful I could get it before Jonesy noticed. It was the only thing that was going to level me out for the next four hours.

I slammed the shot, took a piss, and made it to the first tee just in time. There were no warmup swings, no time to stretch, no nothing. It was as if I were playing a weekend round with my degenerate buddies and not for the biggest purse on the tour. The tour officials were all in attendance at the first tee, and I could feel their cold stares beating down on me while I waited for my turn to hit.

The first swing I put on the ball was piped right down the middle of the fairway. It made zero sense as to why— probably muscle memory. I stumbled when I bent down to pick up my tee, saw stars as the blood rushed away from my brain, and we were off. I parred the first four holes and was doing everything I could to just keep the ball in front of me. There wasn't anything flashy about it: put the ball in play, get on the green, two putt, and get out of there. I figured I'd need to shoot two under to put myself in position. So far, so good. Jonesy couldn't believe what he was seeing. My game had improved since he last saw me, and I mean I did practice, but I was under the influence of something every time I hit golf balls. The golf course was still my sanctuary in a way, but the days of being the kid playing while the grown men drank were long gone.

Jonesy and I made it through the front nine just one-over par. I was managing and feeling better as the day went along. Jonesy and I were also back to being cordial like old times after our icy car ride. I could tell he still held a little resentment, but he saw that I could play a little bit still despite my state of mind and the punishment I was putting my body through.

The good times didn't last, however, and things changed drastically for me on the back nine. I bogeyed the thirteenth and fourteenth holes. On the fifteenth tee, I lost my drive so far right that it landed in some kind of bush. We weren't quite sure what it was, whether it was marked or not, so we didn't play a provisional ball off the tee. One of our playing partners was certain it was a hazard and that we could drop laterally depending on whether we could identify that it was, in fact, my golf ball.

Jonesy knew things were slipping away a bit, and the curse words were flowing steadily out of my mouth. I was tearing myself apart verbally and going down a dark hole that booze would have helped me climb out of, or at least survive in for a few more holes. I didn't have time to make any concoctions for the course. A little vodka in my Gatorade was always the easiest way to hide the booze from the tour officials.

As we got towards the hazard, we could not identify my ball. One of the tour officials who was following along with our play told me that I would have to walk back to the tee to re-hit, and that I should have played a provisional out of caution. It was the last trigger that I needed to come completely unhinged.

Usually, my ire was only directed inward, but this official got the majority of every bad word I ever learned in my life. Jonesy, at one point, had to hold me back from hitting this seventy-year-old gentleman who was just doing what the game required of him.

I worked myself into such a state that I got dizzy, and the walls started to cave in. I threw up all over myself and projectile vomited all over the tour official's shoes. Jake Steadman, ladies and gentlemen... We'll be here all night.

There's nothing to say after my very public meltdown. I put my head down and walked back to the tee. The tirade had drawn the interest of the small crowd and the other players on neighboring holes. Jonesy walked five yards ahead of me and was probably thinking he should have listened to Bri. My attitude and inability to regulate my emotions were on full display. I didn't say another word for the rest of the round and finished with a whimper, ending the day near the bottom of the leaderboard.

After turning in my scorecard, I was asked to meet with the tour officials to discuss my actions from the day. Jonesy said he would come with me, even though I could tell he didn't want to be there. I told him everything was fine, and he could wait outside.

"Mr. Steadman," one of the officials said to me. He was a proper-looking gentleman who outwardly showed he had his stuff together. He was the complete opposite of who I was. "Your actions in most tournaments you play in were brought to our attention before this event. And you were on very thin ice before your little episode today. Craig is one of our longest tenured and most respected officials on this tour, and your behavior was unbecoming of anyone we want representing us."

I could feel the weight of my actions was about to smother me. A sinking feeling developed in my stomach. I was having a hard time catching a deep breath. I wasn't sure if this was death felt like.

"We have made the decision as a governing body to remove you from any and all future tournaments. You will be disqualified for the remainder of this tournament, and you are no longer allowed back on premise at any events from here on out," the man said to me.

The group of officials all packed up their belongings and left me there without a chance to defend myself. I mean there wasn't much defending. I went to the bathroom and looked at myself in the mirror. The bags under my eyes were pronounced. I looked like I hadn't slept in three weeks. The light in my eyes was officially out. I didn't even know who I was looking at anymore and couldn't remember the last time I truly felt anything other than the bottomless pit of despair or the high of a cocaine bender.

Jonesy was waiting out by the car to take my sorry ass home. We didn't say a word to each other the entire ride.

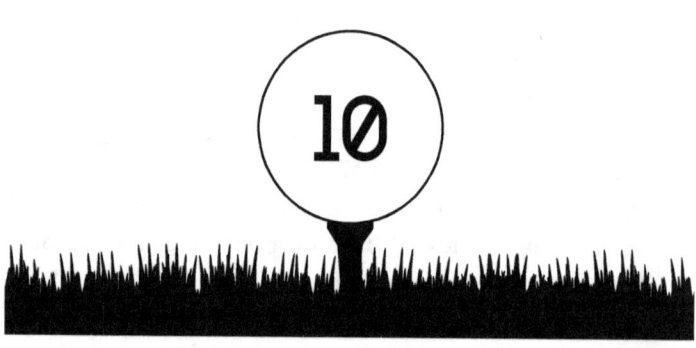

"This is the fucking dumbest rule in golf," Jonesy said. It wasn't often that Jonesy swore, so I could tell the moment meant just as much to him as it did to me.

Before I could look at what he was talking about, it was just nice to hear Jonesy's voice because my brain had warped back to that last moment in the car after I got kicked off the tour. We didn't say a thing on that car ride home, and there weren't many pleasantries shared back and forth before he went back to Massachusetts. It was the last time I heard from him for quite some time.

I finally caught up to Jonesy and peeked at what got him so distraught. All I could do was muster a smirk. My ball did find the fairway. The problem was that my ball also happened to land squarely into a divot.

Golf's number one rule is to play the ball as it lies. Here I was thinking that I hit the fairway and could attack my next shot. Unfortunately, my ball was sitting a few centimeters under the earth in the middle of what felt like a crater. There was no relief from a situation like this. I was not impeded by a sprinkler head or any other man-made object. I was just impeded by some other golfer's gross negligence in repairing the divot they made.

In the past, this was exactly the moment when I lost my composure. This was the mistake that would ultimately end any kind of hope I had for closing out a match. It was also the time I would sneak away to grab a sip of something to calm my nerves. My mouth watered and then dried up very quickly. My heart rate rose as I started thinking about how this ball would react to my club face hitting it.

Trying to make a swing right now in ideal conditions was hard enough. I stared down into the earth and shut my eyes. Finding my breath was the first thing I needed to do.

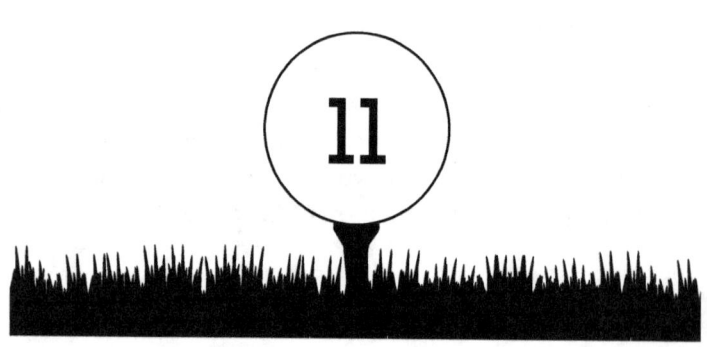

I was jolted awake by the captain announcing we would be making our descent into Boston. It would take us about thirty minutes to land due to other traffic in the area. I must have been asleep for most of the flight. This whole day seemed like a dream sequence.

Bri had called me about ten hours ago this morning to let me know about Jonesy. I still had zero idea of what was going on, and my contacts at home were few and far between. I had no friends outside of Jonesy and my old man, whom I hadn't talked to since I got kicked off the tour several years ago. There was no way to get the most up-to-date information about what exactly I was coming home to while I was sitting on that plane. You could say I was flying blind.

I had no idea if he was alive. All I could do was watch the Massachusetts coastline come into view from the plane's window.

The moments after Bri hung up were a blur. I was still incredibly fucked up, maybe more so than I had ever been in my life. I still wasn't sure the call was real. I walked back towards my couch and sat down for a second to collect myself. The alarm bells were ringing in my head, and the decisions I made the night before were starting to come into view.

The pill bottles. The loaded pistol. The cocaine. The booze. They were all laid out in front of me. I really didn't want to think about what I was planning. All I knew was I had to find my way up to Massachusetts with limited time and resources.

I knocked on my landlord's door. His name was Mike, and he was one of my old man's good friends from the club up in Ridgeway. He was retiring early, just about the time I was thinking of coming down to Florida years ago. He told me I had a place to stay in his back guest house for as long as I wanted it. He and my old man went way back, and Mike had seen Jackie through some very tumultuous times. When he opened the door, he probably had flashbacks of helping out Jackie when times were tough.

Mike let me in and offered me water. He could tell I needed it.

"Jakey, you look like shit kid," Mike said to me in his thick Boston accent. Mike lived the snowbird life and had put up with me for a very long time. I wasn't the best tenant in the world and barely paid him. But he always accepted my life-style and never intervened when I couldn't make the rent.

I felt like a real piece of shit when I asked him if he had any miles or any cash to help me get home. I needed a one-way ticket as quickly as I could, and I had no idea when I would be coming back.

Mike had heard a little bit of information about Jonesy. News travels fast at the club. Apparently, Jonesy got sick very quickly and ended up getting med flighted due to some kind of infection. One day, he was fine, running around with the kids. The next day, he was in Mass General fighting for his life.

"Whatever you need, Jakey," he said.

His generosity still made zero sense to me, and maybe it never would. He didn't want to step in as a figure of authority when I was fucking up my life, but he was always good to me. Mike had a little bit of a checkered past himself and had been sober for a few years now.

"You go home and figure out what is going on. Stay there as long as you need. I'll get your place cleaned up, and it will be here whenever you want to come back," he said.

I did my best to hold back tears. A lump in my throat started to form. He held out his hand and nodded, meaning I didn't have to say a word. When he shook my hand, he also handed me an envelope with money in it. I did all that I could not to break down right there.

I packed as many clothes as I could get into a suitcase. As I went to leave, I looked back and saw the mess that I had left Mike. A professional cleaner would eventually clean up the life that I created down here. It was no life at all. I walked out the door and wasn't sure when I would ever see this place again.

You would have thought losing status on the tour and losing that revenue stream, no matter how small it was, would have been the kick in the ass that I needed to get my shit together. You could say my life went in the complete opposite direction. I caddied anywhere I could get a bag to carry and spent all the cash I made at the bar or the casino or at the strip club later that night. This process played out night after night, day after day, for years. I wasn't even sure how long it lasted because every day was like time traveling. One moment I was fucked up...the next, I was not. Then rinse and repeat to get over the thought of having to live this existence.

In essence, I was leaving nothing behind. No full-time job. No significant other. No real purpose in life. I had thought about coming home many times before. I wasn't even invited to Jonesy's wedding after my stunt the last time I saw him. Bri wouldn't allow me on the guest list despite his willingness to give me a second chance. Bri was a smart woman. She always knew when to make the right call.

I was an embarrassment in every sense of the word, with a self-image that matched the way other people viewed me.

The captain came back on the loudspeaker and asked for the crew to take their seats for landing. All I could do was stare out the window and wonder what would happen next.

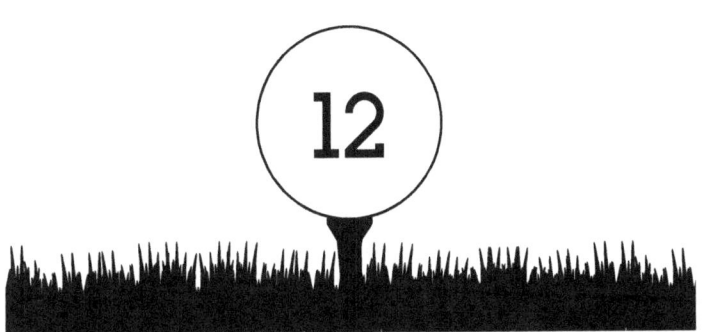

I t's an incredibly powerful image when you see your best friend lying in a hospital bed, breathing tubes sticking out of his face, and the slow beep of machines keeping him alive. The thousand-mile stare I had out the window of the plane was no match for the feeling I had right now.

None of this made sense. Jonesy was the model of health. He ran, ate right, and took care of his body, maybe better than anyone. Sure, he enjoyed the brown liquor occasionally, from what I remembered, but his lifestyle was the complete opposite of mine, and that was usually a good recipe to follow.

Staring at Jonesy, I had this sinking feeling that it should have been me in that bed.

It was exactly twelve hours from when I got the call from Bri to when I arrived home in Boston. I was able to sleep off the mistakes I made from the night before and had it mostly together. I still reeked of my apartment and the stale scent of the disaster it was. I didn't have time to get in the shower or really put myself together. I just knew I needed to get home, and Mike got me on the first flight out of Tampa.

Bri greeted me without a hug or an embrace. She explained that Jonesy may have a fungal infection picked up from his dentist. Apparently, he was in there for a routine cleaning on Thursday morning, and by Saturday, he was in this vegetative state. His lungs were barely holding on, and they had to move fast to get him transported from back home to Mass General to get him to the best doctors in the world. The next twenty-four to seventy-two hours would be incredibly touch-and-go. You could see the stress it was putting on Bri. She hadn't slept a wink. The kids were at home with her parents, forty miles away.

I still had no idea why she called me to come.

"Doctors are going to keep him under for as long as he needs to," Bri said softly. "They are hoping by taking the load off his lungs, the breathing tubes will be able to strengthen them back up and get to a point where he can breathe on his own again."

She looked at Jonesy. I turned my head to look at my friend. Bri's entire life was lying limp in that hospital bed. I couldn't imagine what was going through her head. And all she had at that moment was me, doing my best not to say something stupid to ruin my invite to be by his bedside.

"Whatever you need me to do," is all that I could offer.

She looked at me, unsure of what I was capable of. Nothing else needed to be said.

For the next three days, I did not leave the hospital. People came and went to bring things for Bri and to offer condolences. Some people gave me a once-over and finally realized who I was. We had small talk to discuss life, but nothing of meaning was ever discussed. The one thing I made sure not to do was leave. It felt like the only thing I could do to make up for the years of neglect I thrust upon my friend, especially after embarrassing him on the day I got kicked off the tour.

Bri and I didn't interact much. I sat there and waited until she wanted to talk to me, which didn't really happen. I would get her a coffee or some food from the cafeteria. Mike's wad of cash was starting to get lower and lower every time I used it. I wasn't panicking yet, but I think the hospital staff knew I didn't have anywhere to stay, so they let me crash in the family area. Bri must have put in a good word, which was very much appreciated.

The three days in that hospital were hell. Those first twenty-four hours were the longest I had gone without a substance in my body outside of a cigarette, and things were starting to happen to me. A cold shiver overtook my body on night one, even though it was May and it was warm outside in the greater Boston area. I could feel the pain of my body craving a drink coming on strong. The pounding behind my eyes was getting deeper and deeper, and the only thing that could fix it was a snort of cocaine simultaneously up both nostrils.

Bri could see me struggling. She had bigger things to worry about. It was on the third day, I think, when Bri finally came over to me.

"Jake," she put her hand on my shoulder and woke me up. "I need to ask you a favor."

A favor? This was the first time she had ever asked that of me in the entire time I knew her. "Yeah, what's up?" I said, coming to my senses.

"My parents have the kids and are taking care of everything with them. But they need someone to take Reggie out. He needs to be walked and given dinner tonight. Do you think you can do that for me?" She sounded unsure of the ask herself.

"Yes, sure. I don't have a car..."

Before I could finish my sentence, she was going through her bag.

"You can take mine. It's parked in the visitor lot down the street. It's a red Volvo. I'm on the second floor. Just hit the security button, and it should go off. Here's our address. She'd had all this prepared. Bri must have been a very good mom. The type who had a snack or a piece of candy at the ready when her kid got a little cranky.

"Reggie's food is in the fridge. Can you stay at the house and take him out in the morning? There's a couch in the basement. You can crash down there and make yourself at home."

That last part surprised us both.

"Yeah...yeah sure. I'll take care of it. Reggie is a dog, right?" I asked.

"Yes, our golden retriever. Feel free to take him out for a long walk. I'm sure he's been cooped up with my parents and the kids."

This was the first time Bri had ever asked anything of me, and I sure as shit wasn't going to fuck it up. Jonesy had made it through the seventy-two-hour window, and they were just waiting for the right time to bring him out of his induced coma. The worst was hopefully behind us, and Bri had to start thinking about putting the pieces back together for when her family would eventually all be home.

I took the keys and headed south. It was the first time I'd headed that way in a very long time.

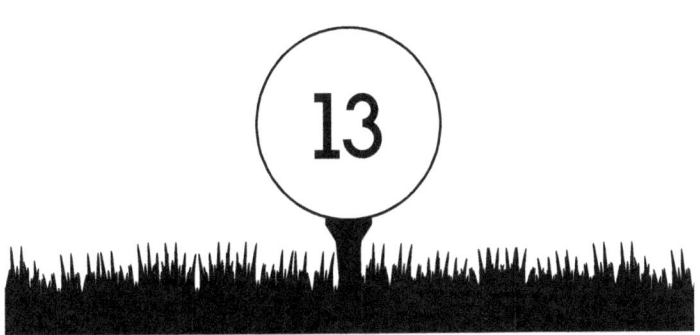

"We're going to be okay, bud," Jonesy said. His voice was weak. He could only move his arm a few inches off the bed to take my hand. His eyes were the only other thing on his body that could move in my direction as I sat by his bedside.

It had been a full week since the doctors put Jonesy in a coma to try to speed up his recovery. I had been going back and forth to take care of Reggie every single day and would drive back up to Boston to be there for whatever Bri needed. Our interactions weren't much. But I was there. When she told me Jonesy would be taken off life support and woken up on that seventh day, my shoulders dropped with such relief it was as if a 100-pound gorilla finally hopped off my back. This was the first time I had cared about someone else in a very long time. I guess I didn't realize how much stress was building inside of me, not just from this ordeal, but from my entire life.

The week at Jonesy's house was not easy for me. When I first arrived back in the town I had left behind, I was still an absolute mess. The first few nights in the hospital were rough, but that week at Jonesy's house was some of the worst pain I've ever felt in my life. I had heard of addicts who would be dope sick and would relapse in those first few days due to the physical pain their bodies were going through and due to a lack of substance of choice.

There were no words to describe the amount of sweat that had come out of my body in the middle of the night at Jonesy's. In the moments I did get some rest, the nightmares would alarm me so much that it was better to just stay up and lie there with my eyes open. My mind kept going back to the scene that played out in my apartment when I woke up to Bri's phone call. The taste of steel from the end of the gun was something I couldn't get out of my mouth. I still wasn't sure whether it actually happened or if it was some kind of dream sequence that just felt all too real, like the ones where you dream you are falling, and your body jolts awake like the floor is no longer beneath you.

Reggie stayed close to me every single night. He must have known something was up. He also must have been just as confused, wondering where his rightful owners were and why this stranger was oozing out sweat like a flu patient.

The temptations in Jonesy's house were always there. The scotch collection he had in his kitchen was rather robust and delicious-looking. The local watering holes I passed on the ride home were always beckoning. One night, I even went into the bar and ordered a beer but left it right there on the table in front of me. The willpower it took to not get up in the middle of the night and end the leg cramps and pain in my abdomen with just one swig of Johnnie Walker Black was something I hadn't even realized I possessed, because saying no to things wasn't really my strongpoint, especially when it came to getting fucked up. But, I knew the alternative was to never see my friend again. I'm sure Bri, as much as she needed my help, was scared shitless about what Jonesy's loser friend was doing to her home in their absence.

It took Jonesy a few days to regain the strength to start moving around in his bed. Watching him move like a ninety-year-old after hip surgery made me realize this was going to be a long haul for him. The doctors were just starting to pinpoint what had happened and what the best course of action was for getting him back to as close to 100 percent as possible.

His lungs had started to fill with fluid due to this infection, and without the power of those machines, he would have been dead. Bri and Jonesy were just lucky they didn't mess around and got him the care he needed immediately. Things would have looked a lot different without that early intervention.

The back-and-forth to Boston continued for me as the kids stayed with Bri's parents. She never left that hospital once. I had to break it to Bri that my funds were low, and she handed over her credit card to make sure I could get gas in the car and Reggie the food that he needed. She even told me to go food shopping for myself. I felt ashamed and embarrassed that I could not contribute.

Either Bri had softened on me over the last few weeks, or she just didn't have time to fight that battle. I was gaining new empathy for Bri and Jonsey's situation. Putting others ahead of my stupid needs was new for me, but I knew I would do anything for Bri, just like I would for my best friend. If she needed me as well, there was no doubt that this new version of Jake was going to be there.

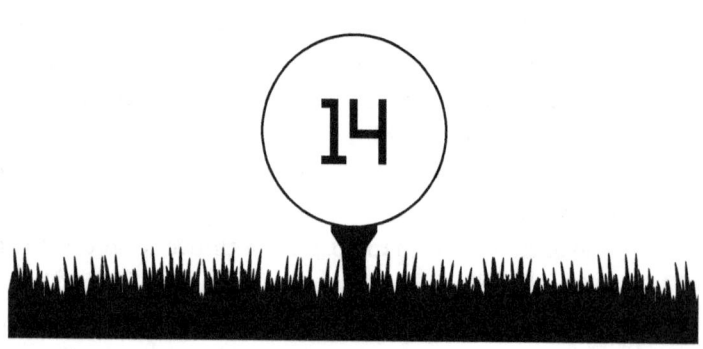

Jonesy's health came back as the days and weeks went on. He was the model of good health before, and the doctors agreed that his fitness is not only what kept him alive, but what would help him bounce back to an eventual full recovery. Any weaker person wouldn't have been as lucky. Death certainly would have come for me. An uncrowded funeral would have been my fate.

I could sense my time was coming to an end up here, and at some point, I would have to head back down to Florida to figure out what to do next with my life. I hadn't touched a drink since I landed in Boston. It was the longest I had gone since I was sixteen years old without getting fucked up in some fashion. I drank or smoked or did drugs for half of my existence. It was something that gave me the chills the more time I spent sober. Being a drunk and drug user certainly wasn't a label I wanted to live with anymore.

Bri had planned to get the kids, her parents, and Jonesy's parents together to celebrate having their family under one roof for the first time since this nightmare happened. It was a small event without much fanfare, and I was invited, but I felt a little out of place. I didn't want to be anywhere else, though. If I were being honest, this house was starting to feel like home.

It was nice to connect with Jonesy's mom and dad. We never really had much of a relationship outside of golf. Jonesy's dad and my old man knew each other from the club, but knowing how he looked at me and how he never asked how Jack was doing, I could sense Jonesy's dad was probably in the indifferent crowd about my father.

I could see the internal struggle Jonesy was having as the man of the house. It was all over his face. Men fight silent battles, and this one was Jonesy's right now. It was supposed to be him who cared for his family, and not the other way around. He was a proud man. He wasn't a macho man or someone who oozed masculinity, but he cared about his family and cared about being healthy. You could tell he inherently cared that his condition prevented him from being the person he worked so hard to be.

With the kids in bed and the party winding down, I helped clean off the dishes and put things away tidily into the dishwasher. This was a far cry from the remnants of disaster that I had left in Florida at my apartment. I couldn't remember the last time I cared for anything, let alone washed a dish. When I was on my own, my sole purpose was waiting for my next opportunity to get completely obliterated.

Jonesy had to use a cane to get around, but he somehow managed to sneak up behind me, masked behind the sound of the running water.

"I never thought I'd see the day," he said with a laugh. Jonesy still had a way to lighten the mood or crack a positive joke despite his condition.

He put his hand on my shoulder. I kept my head down and kept on with the dishes.

"Bri told me what you've done the last few weeks," he said. "I just want to..."

"You don't have to..." I interrupted.

He went to say something and stopped his thought. It was my turn to speak.

"I'm sorry, man," I said with tears welling up in my eyes,

my focus on the last plate fading. "What I did to you the last time I saw you, and how long it's been. I just…" I took a long pause. "I'm just so glad you're still here."

Expressing emotions wasn't my thing. Jonesy grabbed me by the back of the neck, and we embraced. I didn't have a brother, but this is what one of those hugs felt like. It was like, in that moment, the damage of the past was all forgotten. We had an opportunity to move forward and rebuild this relationship. For the first time, I could potentially do this sober and as a changed person. I hoped Jonesy felt the same way.

"I'll make arrangements to get out of your hair as quickly as I can," I said, pulling away from the hug and using the sleeves of my shirt to dry my eyes.

Jonesy made a motion as if to say that doesn't need to be discussed right now.

"I just got to reach out to Mike and let him know I'll be coming home."

I finished up the last plate and headed downstairs to give him time to hang out with his wife.

Reggie came and nestled up next to me on the pull-out. Dogs are funny creatures. His owner was home, but his routine recently was to come down here and be with me. I don't think he realized how much I appreciated it in that moment.

I wish this had never happened for Jonesy and his family, but even I couldn't deny what it had done for my life to get out of Florida and see things differently. I felt guilty about feeling this way, but having had separation from what I was doing to myself and time to think about where my life was going was the blessing I desperately needed. There wouldn't have been a support system for me if I got sick or hurt. There certainly would not be a long line of people dropping off food to anyone if I were to leave this earth. All these feelings were incredibly heavy. This was usually when I'd turn to drugs or alcohol to numb these feelings, but I wanted to feel them now. Every emotion. It made me feel more alive than any line that ever went up my nose.

I sat there staring at the wall, and Reggie jolted up and ran towards the stairs.

Bri was coming down the steps by herself. Reggie gave her a warm welcome, and she gave a tap on the wall to get my attention, even though I knew she was there.

"Hey Jake, you up?" Bri said. The last month was taxing on Jonesy, but Bri took the brunt of the shit show. She was managing her kids and her life from the hospital. Her parents would bring the kids up when they weren't in school. But Bri didn't want their two daughters to see their father in the shape that he was in, just in case it was the last memory they would have of him. At six and four years old, they were old enough that they were just starting to figure this life out, but still young enough that they did not need a taste of what it's really like out there.

"Yup, I'm here," as I shuffled my body to stand up and speak to her.

"I was wondering if you could come with me," she said and walked towards a closed door in the basement.

In the time that I was in Jonesy's house, I didn't explore outside of the kitchen, the bathroom, and my living quarters on the couch. I treated their house like a museum and wanted to leave zero trace that I was in it. It was the first time I respected anything in probably twenty years.

Bri reached for the top of the door frame and retrieved a key from her tiptoes. She put the key into the lock. She pushed open the door and turned the light on. It was Jonesy's office. There was a computer desk and a shrine to golf littered all over the walls. Flags from all the best courses he had played covered the left wall. A poster of the chip shot Tiger Woods hit on the sixteenth hole at Augusta hung behind the desk. I loved that moment too.

As I was looking around at Jonesy's memories, I felt a numbness that I wasn't part of any of this over the last decade. We had talked about playing all these courses together when we were junior golfers, but life had other plans for me.

Not for Jonesy. He followed through, unsurprisingly, on the things he wanted to do with the game. He just had a different priority around it. He had learned to have fun with the game, which is something I never really did. I only felt something when I succeeded at the game and was given praise or guilt from my father accordingly. Looking at how Jonesy celebrated the game like he did in his office gave me a feeling in my chest that maybe my approach had been all wrong.

I panned the room from left to right and stopped short when I saw his computer. My breath caught, and I could feel a stinging in my eyes for the second time that night. I wasn't sure I would be able to hold back the tears in front of Bri this time. Next to Jonesy's computer were a handful of pictures – one of him and Bri on their wedding day, two pictures of him holding his two girls on the day they were born, and finally a picture of Jonesy and me in a tournament at Ridgeway when we were thirteen years old. The two of us were holding up our trophies with huge smiles on our faces. I had won the junior tournament for the fourth straight year, and Jonesy had finally made it to the winner's circle with a third-place finish. I could replay that day like it was yesterday. It was amazing to share that moment after I saw how hard he had worked that whole summer. He had tried to keep up with me, with how much I was practicing, but his dad actually made him go home from the club and try other sports.

But that was the year he finally broke through.

The smiles on our faces were ear-to-ear. We were two scrawny kids with clothes that looked two sizes too big for us. We were kids having the time of our lives. I picked up the photo and couldn't hold back my emotion.

After all this time, he still held that memory close. As close to him as his own family. I don't even know where anything from my past was. Probably somewhere stuffed in a box in that shitty existence in Florida.

"He loves that picture," Bri said.

I had forgotten Bri was standing there in the room with me.

"It was a special day for both of us," I said, not moving my eyes from this version of myself I had long forgotten existed. I looked really happy. It would only be a year later that my trouble on the golf course began, and the joy that I had in that moment would vanish. It was like the final snapshot of a happy life. I caught a bit of my reflection in the picture frame staring back at me. These two people weren't the same.

"He always told me you were very good. When he came home from Florida that last time, he was crushed," Bri said.

I slowly put the picture down and turned my attention to Bri.

"I had never seen him like that. He didn't talk much, and for the first time, I could sense that he felt he had lost you forever. I tried to tell him that it was a bad idea. I wanted to protect him. He protects me all of the time, and in that moment, I tried to return the favor. But he went anyway, and he was just so disappointed when he got home," she continued.

I was starting to feel very small. The last time I remember feeling like this was on the day they booted me from the tour. If I had to put a name to how I felt, it was shame. I was ashamed of who I had been and even more embarrassed that I could not see the error in my ways.

"It was my call not to invite you to our wedding. He hadn't heard from you and wasn't sure what state you were in. I couldn't let him go through what he went through when he came back the last time he saw you. Especially on our wedding day. I know he had a great time, but something was missing for him."

"We did make a promise that if anything were to happen to him that I would have to call you. It's a promise I didn't think in a million years I would have to make good on," she said, holding back tears.

"I almost didn't do it. But I knew that if he did pull through and you weren't there, that a piece of the trust between us would be gone."

So that answered the question that I had about why she called.

"You stepped up, Jake. He never stopped believing in you, and now I can see why. There's a good person inside of you, and it took me some time to see it. What you did for my family will never be forgotten."

I nodded; words were still not something I could put together.

"I want you to do me a favor," she said. I had no idea how strong of a person Bri was until this whole ordeal. I could see why Jonesy loved her.

"Sure. Anything," was all I could muster.

"I want you to stay," she said.

The gravity of her words hit in a way that I maybe had never felt before. They were motivating and deflating all at the same time. Someone who I thought hated me had changed her tune and all it took was stepping outside myself for a little bit. I was shocked and grateful at the same time. The thought of going back to Florida had been on my mind for some time now.

"I want you to stay and do something else, not for me, but for Jonesy and for yourself. You see that kid in that photo. He's still in there. When Jonesy did eventually talk about you, he mentioned how good you were playing. He said your talent was always there. I want you to stay, and I want you to find that again," she said.

I wasn't completely sure what I was hearing. Playing golf had been so far from my mind for so long, but something shifted when I saw that photo and received Bri's blessing. It was like the sign I never knew I needed.

"Jonesy told me you always used to play the game of golf for other people. Mostly, he shared that you used to play for your dad. What you need, Jake, is to play for that kid in the photo. Jonesy always believed in you. Now, believe in yourself and make a life up here. You can stay as long as you want. We are going to need way more help, and I can't ask my sisters or Jonesy's sisters. They have young families, and our parents are getting old. If you stay, you don't have to pay rent or do anything other than find something you're passionate about. And we all know what that is."

I didn't know what to say.

"Now go out there and prove Jonesy right," Bri demanded and gave me a hug. It was the first embrace we had. I remember the first time I saw her in the hospital a few weeks ago. She was hesitant to have him in the room. Her body language screamed it, and now here we were discussing how I would continue to be a part of her and her family's life.

I looked back at the photo of me and Jonesy. It was as if my younger self was staring straight through my soul. Bri was giving me a ticket to my next chapter, and staring into the eyes of my younger self, I knew I had to take it to save not just myself, but the kid in the photo. He needed me, and for the first time, I felt like it was my responsibility to follow through.

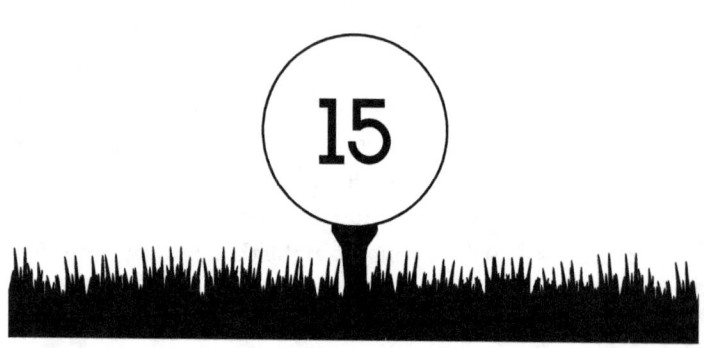

My attention came back to my ball, cratered in the divot. I could tell Jonesy was saying something to me, but I was lost in my search for breath. I was trying to center myself right there on the eighteenth fairway.

"We're going to be okay, bud," I finally said out loud, not exactly sure if I was saying this to Jonesy or myself. They were also the exact words that Jonesy had first said to me in Mass General when he first woke up from his coma.

The irony of it all felt weird. Even Jonesy looked like he was feeling a strange sense of déjà vu.

The truth was, things were going to be just fine no matter what the outcome of this was. The last year of working with Tom and working on myself allowed me to start seeing the long game and finding my way back to life.

The fact that my ball was in this divot was just another bump in the road.

All I could do was laugh and remember the first time Tom had entered my life to teach me about the game of golf.

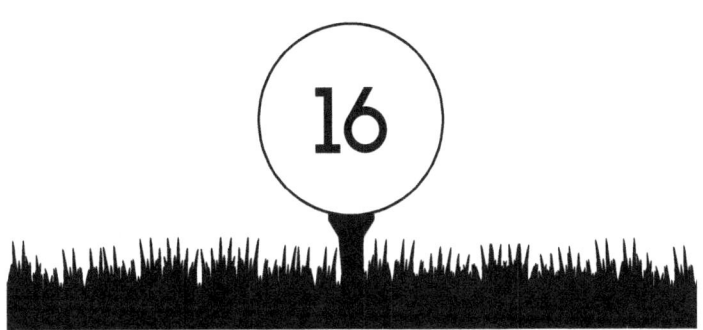

16

I agreed to stay, and Jonesy was thrilled. He was also in desperate need of another capable set of hands in the house to help him with physical therapy and some of the everyday chores of life that were difficult for him to manage at the moment.

Bri's orders were for me to find something that I loved. The only thing I knew in life was golf. I got on the phone with Mike and asked if he would ship my clubs up. I told him I would pay him back.

"No reason to, kid," he told me. "They will be there in the next day or so."

Mike had become my guardian angel over the years. His calmness was always something I appreciated. I knew he had to go through hell to attain that level of Zen, and I was starting to understand where he was coming from after my sobriety carried on.

I didn't go the route of AA or other meetings. Instead, I focused on keeping my promise to my friend and his family that I wouldn't mess up this opportunity and wouldn't go backwards in life ever again. Purpose is a funny thing. When you are without it, the world kind of stops. It's harder to get out of bed. It's harder to make decisions about who you are and what you want to be. But when a man gets just a little taste of what could be, there's a thirst for more that develops inside of him. It's hard to describe fully, but when you believe there's more to life, and go out and act with that belief in mind, you start to build momentum towards your goals, and it was actively building inside of me. Even on the hard days. When my clubs arrived, Mike had left a note inside the bag.

"Give Jonesy my best and have fun swinging these again."

Mike had also loaded me up with some clothes, golf shoes, and a bunch of golf balls to get me going. There was also another wad of cash in the big pocket of the golf bag. I couldn't say thank you enough to Mike. Whenever things got hard, I would think of all the things that Mike had done for me. His love gave me purpose.

"Look what the cat dragged in," Steve Hickey called in my direction as I walked in through the doors of the Clark Center. Steve and I played some junior golf together, and I had heard that he was working his way up through the PGM program to be a head golf professional. He was a decent player and one of the kids who heard about my prowess at Ridgeway but never saw me follow through. By the time I had met Steve, my nosedive into the period where I couldn't get over the hump on the course was in full swing.

It was humbling to ask Steve for a job in exchange for a membership. He said he had a couple of night shifts available if that worked for me. I told him I didn't need to get paid. I just needed to have Clark's as a place where I could practice during the day and not dip too deep into the cash that Mike had sent my way.

We shook hands and he showed me around. The place hadn't changed in twenty years, but it still had everything you could need. There was a gym with golf-specific training machines all over the place. There were two practice greens for chipping and putting, and most importantly indoor and outdoor hitting bays that were open year-round. That meant no matter what the weather, I had no excuse but to get out here and get my groove back.

I was relieved that there was no one around to witness my first bucket of balls. My brain knew exactly what I wanted to do. My body, however, didn't seem to receive the message. I was no longer the skinny kid from the picture on Jonesy's desk. I wasn't even myself from a few years ago when I was still playing decent golf despite my alcohol and drug dependency.

I started with some half shots and immediately tinkered with my grip and my stance after every single swing. This was my normal routine. It's what I knew. There was nobody else around, but I had this sneaking suspicion that there was a set of eyes on me. I could feel it, but I didn't know where it was coming from.

I hit balls for an hour and was completely gassed. Honestly, I was out of energy halfway through the session, but hitting the driver as hard as I could was starting to feel therapeutic. It was as if something was leaving my body with every swing. There were duck hooks and pushed shots all over the place. There were also some dead on the screws. A true mixed bag. I stuck with it and pushed through until I couldn't swing anymore.

I told Steve that I would be there tomorrow and asked what time my shift started later in the week.

"Get here at three p.m.," he said while occupied with a customer in the shop.

I walked out of Clark's still unable to shake the feeling that someone was keeping an eye on me.

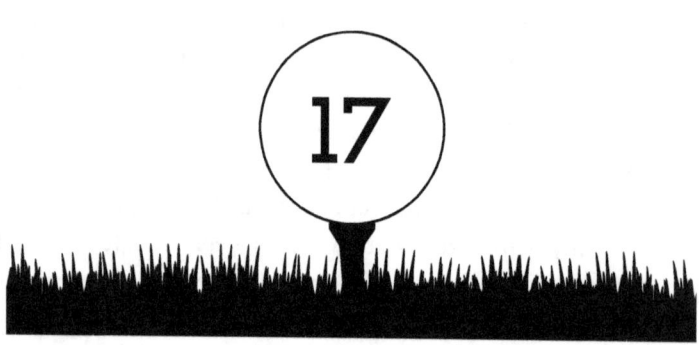

17

"Jake," Steve poked his head into the backroom while I washed golf balls I had just picked from the range. Clark's usually got packed in the evening, and I was the only thing standing between golfers and their stress relief after a long day. I shut the machine off to hear what Steve had to say.

"The old man wants to see you after your shift. Are you good with that?" Steve asked.

I had this sense of panic that he was talking about my old man. I had been up in our hometown for almost a month and a half and hadn't said a word to him about my presence back home. I knew he knew. It was a small town after all. But for my sobriety's sake, I decided to keep my distance and focus on things that I could control, like helping Jonesy get to his appointments, taking Reggie outside for our morning walk, and keeping up with my daily ritual of finding my golf game.

"Sure thing," I said. Knowing that Steve didn't know my old man all that well, other than what he witnessed when we were kids, I realized that he was, in fact, talking about Tom Clark, the legendary teacher at the facility bearing his name.

I had no idea what Tom wanted with me. I was a part-timer who kept to myself and worked on my game. Nonetheless, I kept my word and went and saw him towards the end of my shift. It was later than usual for Tom to still be on property. I walked towards his barn, where he taught his students daily. It was like a revolving door of golfers coming in and out of his laboratory. Many came out with smiles on their faces. Others were perplexed by the teachings, still unsure how to put together the wisdom that Tom was trying to impart on them.

I walked around the front side of his open garage door to the barn and saw him watching the TV mounted on the wall. He was rocking back and forth and didn't acknowledge my entrance. The room itself was a shrine to the game of golf. Pictures of Ben Hogan and other legends covered the walls. There were clubs and gadgets all over the place. There was even an axe leaning against the wall in the corner. It kind of reminded me of Jonesy's office.

I went to speak and was quickly interrupted.

"You see that right there," he said, never breaking his gaze at the TV. I had no idea if he even knew I was in the room. 'That right there is speed. He's going to be a hell of a player."

I realized this was a listening meeting. So, I kept my mouth shut.

"You're a fixer. You always have been, I bet. It's just what you do," Tom said. Again, he didn't make eye contact, but this time I knew he was addressing me directly.

I suddenly realized that the feeling of being watched was, in fact, Tom Clark keeping tabs on me. The way I practiced must have driven him crazy. Every time something didn't go my way, I tried to create a new feel and simply hit the ball on the center of the club face. That's what happens when you don't actually learn your golf swing and just try to take on the game yourself. I had no direction or true understanding of how to practice correctly.

"You're an athlete, so you've got that going for you. And you've got talent," he said as he rose to his feet out of the rocking chair. "But you've got no idea how to swing the club." He was now making direct eye contact with me. A hulking figure he was not, but his words carried weight. And he was blunt. I liked "blunt." It was the first time anyone had the balls to be so straightforward with me. I knew what he was talking about and, already, I felt myself starting to shrink at the thought of whatever critique was coming next, but I was intrigued.

"How good do you want to be?" Tom asked.

"I haven't really thought too much about it," that was a lie. The truth was, ever since Bri threw down the gauntlet, I knew I wanted to compete again at a very high level. What level? I had no idea. My brain was feeling great, and my body, as horrible as it looked in my eyes, was starting to remember the things I self-taught myself on the golf course.

"Are you willing to work at this?" Tom said, breaking my mini daydream.

This moment felt like a reset in my life. I hadn't answered Tom yet, but when I honestly thought about this question, I remembered the little kid from that picture. I remember the kid who would spend all his free time at Ridgeway and practice from sunup to sundown. I remember the love I had in those moments and thought about how Jonesy developed a love for the game in a different way. If I could find a way to have fun and drive towards a goal, then that, to me, was winning. That was worth living out a dream for me.

"I am, sir," I said with conviction. I was liking this version of myself. The one who showed up for others. The one who showed up for himself. The one who said something and meant it and held eye contact with people. It was my word, and it was starting to mean something.

"Good," Tom said. "Let's get to work."

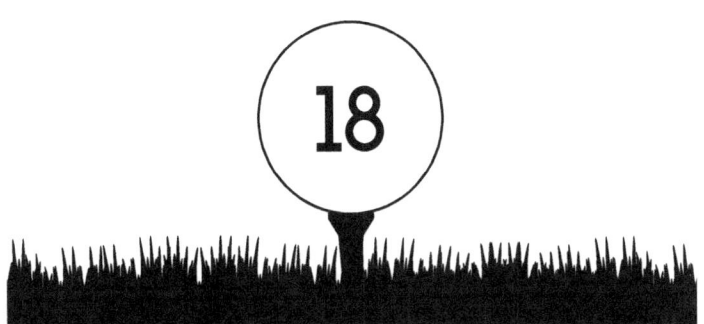

18

I could barely make out what the guy behind the counter was saying to me. This was the third or fourth day in a row without sleep or a meal. I had completely lost count at this point. The bender I was on was coming to an end. I was in line at the sporting goods store to make sure of it.

"This one right here is a real beauty," the salesman said. "Great for personal protection and keeping your family safe."

He held up the handgun and placed it on the counter. It was my first time ever buying a weapon.

"You look like a good man," he said. "Just fill out this paperwork and you can pick it up in three days after a background check."

His voice remained kind of fuzzy, but when he said I was a good man, I knew he had no idea who I was. I signed the papers and paid for my new purchase in cash. Then I went and found my way back to the bar.

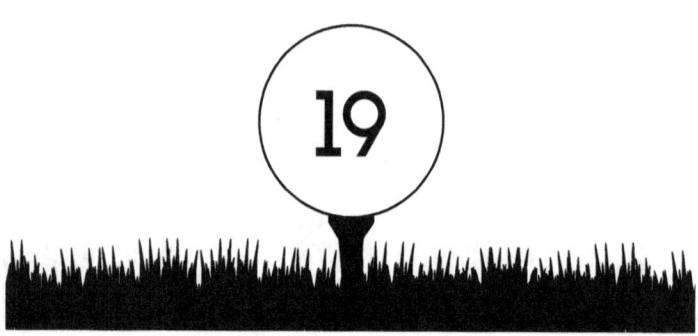

19

"Take the club in your left hand and hit little chip shots," Tom demanded.

I had been playing golf my entire life and had never done this before. It almost seemed remedial. But here I was, asking for a complete reset, so I had to accept whatever teachings came my way.

Trying to perform this little drill that seemed beneath me was one of the most humbling experiences in my life. The club would go back, and I would shank a ball to the right. I would chunk the next one and blade one on a line drive. All Tom wanted was the club to make the ball go a few feet in front of me with good solid contact on the center of the face. I couldn't do that. Not once.

"Now take the club in your right hand and hit little chip shots," Tom said.

I was already embarrassed as it was, so the humiliation would most likely continue. Here I was thinking that I could be a good golfer again and hitting a chip shot with one hand was the most impossible task. I worried that this failure would lead to frustrations that could derail me before I even got started.

I took the club in my right hand fully expecting to fail. This time, I didn't.

"Good," Tom said.

An inner sigh of relief eased through me. That small bit of positive reinforcement was all that I needed. It was something that was earned and not something that was imagined. I accomplished the task and continued to lay the club on the back of the ball without much effort.

"We have figured out something," Tom smiled. "We know that you have never trained your left hand or arm to do what it needs to do in a golf swing."

I knew I was about to get a master's in the physics of swinging the golf club. The simple joy of making a ball hit the center of the club face and move forward ten feet was exhilarating. I wanted more of it. Maybe success was my new drug of choice.

As the days and weeks passed, the lessons progressed. It probably looked funny to everyone else on the range that I was only hitting one-handed chips for the majority of my early practice. I could have cleaned up the balls one by one with how far they were going in front of me. But I was teaching myself to feel for what my arms and hands were supposed to do in the golf swing.

Instead of trying to fix myself every single swing, Tom just wanted me to focus on this task. That was it. "Keep it simple and keep it consistent" were his main messages. Rotate my arms and rotate them through.

Every time I got comfortable, I would start trying to hit full shots and get frustrated.

"Don't skip steps," Tom would say. It was that amount of accountability that I had always needed, and I let it burn deeper into my muscle memory with every swing. Skipping steps had been part of my daily life for ages, so I needed to be patient with myself and give full attention to the task ahead of me. Not living in the moment and thinking ahead to the outcome, both positive and negative, but mostly negative, is something that developed in my teens. It was like a curse that was cast over me after that first bout of failure. I had nobody to tell me to keep it simple. I just had someone telling me that I wasn't doing enough, without giving me the road map to point me in the right direction.

The days turned to weeks, and the weeks turned to months. The urge to return to my old life was almost completely gone. There were always going to be moments when the easy road of relapse felt tempting. But the hard path I was putting myself through, willingly, of course, was always more worth it.

While I was finding my stride, Jonesy was slowly returning to full health. He was working again, part-time from home, and had the strength to pick up his kids and walk the dog. The mornings were for Reggie, Jonesy, and me. We talked about life. We talked about recovery. We sometimes didn't say anything at all. It was like we were in sync again, just like when we were twelve years old. Both of us opened up to each other like we never had before, and I realized we were fighting similar battles but with completely different circumstances.

"Do you think I could come to some of your lessons?" Jonesy asked one morning on our walks. "It would mean a lot to me, and I'd love to be back around the game."

I liked the thought of that very much. I remember how Bri mentioned he saw some things in my game that he had never seen before when I was in Florida. So, something was working when I had the reins myself. Now that Tom and a clean bill of health were running the show, it probably didn't hurt to have someone in my corner who knew me and my game. Jonesy worked hard at everything that he did. He grinded at his life, his career, at fatherhood, and at recovery from the illness more than anyone I had ever met. Having that in my corner would have to rub off in some capacity.

"Let me ask Tom," I said. "But I'd very much appreciate it." I could tell he appreciated it, too.

"How are the lessons going?" Jonesy asked as he picked up a stick and threw it for Reggie. Reggie darted off down the path behind the house and disappeared from sight.

"Honestly, they're going great," I said. "I've lost confidence so many times throughout the process, but Tom has a way of making me stick with it. Every time I'm ready to give up, something clicks, and I manage to make the proper adjustments. I really wish I had this when I was a kid, Jonesy. Who knows what my life would be like now?"

Jonesy nodded.

"Can I ask you a question?" he said. I could tell this one would be deep. After his illness, Jonesy sometimes got into the mood to think a little more philosophically.

"How far do you want to take this?" he asked.

It was a great question, and one I'd heard from both him and Tom by now. Golf was something that I did, and that was about it. My dad was the one with the dreams and aspirations for how far I could take the game. I just fell in line. But in this new phase of my life, the question felt heavy with meaning and possibility, like it wasn't even really about the golf. It was more about how far I wanted to take myself on this journey.

"I don't know, Jonesy," I said playfully. "I think I'm ready to qualify for the U.S. Open!" I said this with a laugh, but it really wasn't that far out of the realm of possibility to take the next eight to nine months to practice and keep my handicap low enough for the qualifier. The actual qualifier wasn't that far from the house, and people do it every year just to see how their game stacks up. Who knows? Maybe I'd catch lightning in a bottle.

"I'm there," Jonesy said. His tone shook the playfulness of the moment. He was making eye contact with me and there was nothing playful in his stare.

"If you go for it then I will be your caddie," he said.

Jonesy was definitely making gains with his health, but to carry a bag for eighteen holes seemed out of the question. Maybe he needed something to work for just as much as I did. I looked him dead in the eyes and shook his hand.

We both had something to shoot for over the next few months. Two friends, going after a dream. Just like the old days.

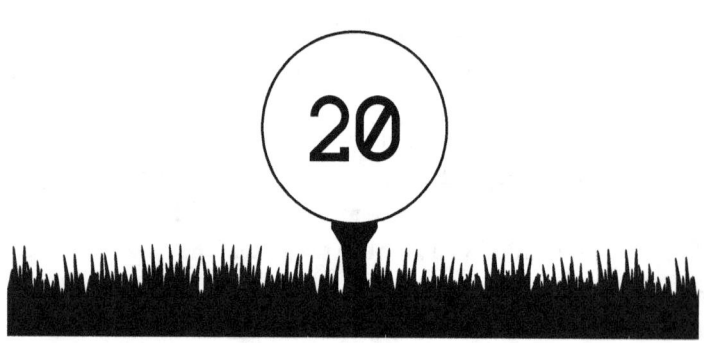

I told Tom about my deal with Jonesy at practice later that day. He leaned back in his rocking chair and mulled over the proposition.

"Sounds fun, kid," Tom said. "We've got a lot of work to do."

Tom had gotten my swing back to a place where I could find some consistency. When I went out for practice rounds, I would consistently shoot in the seventies and flirt with the occasional level par round. Some of my old habits would come up late, and the scores would balloon on the final few holes, but I wasn't bringing the old attitude I had with me. I let these things happen and would get back to work the next day.

Apparently, Tom's idea of fun differed from mine, and his goal over the next few months was to do psychological warfare on me while on the course. Jonesy would drive a cart next to me while I walked during my practice rounds, keeping a close eye on how I handled certain situations.

Tom would hide in the woods where my ball would land and kick a perfectly placed drive down the middle of the fairway into the tall rough. Sometimes he would take my ball altogether, throw it out of play, and say that I was hitting four from the spot as if I was playing a penalty shot off the tee.

All of it was to get a place where it would potentially piss me off. I knew what he was doing. He wanted to see the old me come out. I tried and tried to block that out. Some days were better than others. If I limited damage to my scorecard on that hole, he would take it easier on me. If I fucked up, then who knows what his next scheme would be.

His favorite thing to do, however, was to take my drive and plop it right in the middle of a divot. The bigger the crater, the better for him. I used to think that he would go out and make some of his own, just to know that he would have a juicy one waiting for me when I walked up the fairway to find my ball.

He didn't discriminate. Some were filled with sand. Some were filled with half turf and half sand. Some were clearly from hacks who had no idea how to shallow out the club on the way down and would take half of the Earth with them.

Tom was a bit of a masochist when it came to golf, and I could tell he enjoyed it. Secretly, I was enjoying it too.

What he did do was teach me how to hit the shot that was needed for the situation. Every time he put me in positions to fail, he would teach me how to succeed. I wasn't alone on the golf course with Jonesy there to keep a watchful eye on me and Tom was there to fill my thought bank up with positive memories of making par or better from really shit lies.

Tom was preparing me for every possible outcome on the course. My game was improving, and when he told me to enter a few local tournaments to get myself ready for golf, where every shot counted, I fared pretty well. Each time I played, I improved. I was playing myself into contention, and every time we went out to practice, the stakes were higher.

It was like Tom knew this level of training was exactly what I needed, almost like he could see into the future.

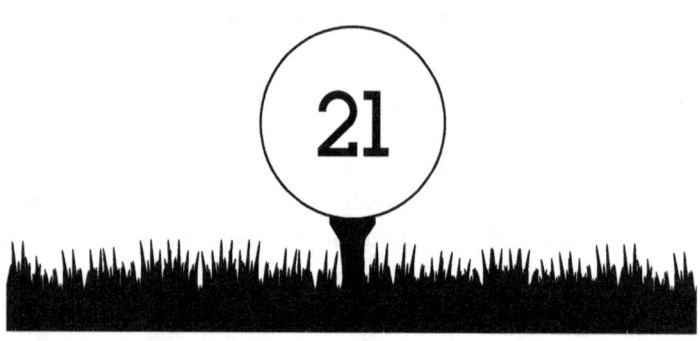

Jonesy wasn't wrong. Getting penalized for hitting a fairway is such a shitty rule. I immediately started to play out the scenarios of what this ball would do coming out of this hole in the ground.

The ball was in the front part of the divot. I could get the club on the back of the ball, but there was no way that thing would generate any spin. I had 184 yards to the pin and needed about 179 to clear a bunker that protected the green. The green was elevated and small, typical of the New England region. Playing in the front bunker wasn't the worst idea in the world. But with everything on the line and needing to get up and down, I wasn't sure I was comfortable doing it. Factoring in the crowd that was forming with the news that I was in position for one of the final spots also made the idea of having to play a clean bunker shot with everyone watching massively daunting.

The play was to carry the bunker and just hope it would slow down enough to make my chip shot coming back easier. The green sloped from back to front severely, so there was nothing easy about the chip shot. But my back would be to the crowd, and I could focus on just hitting the green and letting the slope do with it what it wanted.

"What's the pin, Jonesy?" I asked. My concentration was still down on the ball. Luckily, there wasn't a ton of mud on it that would send it in any direction it wanted.

"It's eighty-four to the stick. We need 179 to cover that bunker," Jonesy said. He looked down at the ball, too. "You playing long?"

I liked how Jonesy and I were in lockstep. It was something that I really needed in that moment. Having Jonesy as my main support in a sport that puts you on an island to fend for yourself when push came to shove made it feel less daunting. The play was to take enough club to carry the bunker and let the outcome be what it was, without getting upset.

I took a slow breath. "Give me the six."

I knew a five iron would be tough to keep the ball in the air, but my six iron was a club I trusted in situations like this. I knew that I could get enough on it. Plus, the adrenaline of the moment would give me a few extra yards that I had to account for.

The moment was now.

I studied the green in the distance and started to pick out a line. I was happy people were up there, so I could pick one person to focus on and just try to hit it directly at them. I had no idea who the guy in the purple shirt was, but I might thank him later for letting me think about drilling him with my approach shot.

I took a deep breath. The entire tournament was most likely riding on this shot. Everyone around the green or behind me lining the fairways had no idea that I had found trouble in the fairway. This was on me and Jonesy to figure out.

I focused on my guy in purple and came back to the ball, mentally thanking Tom for making my life difficult during the training. I rotated both of my arms back and followed through. The contact on the back of the ball was clean. But a little too clean. In a perfect world, a clean lie would have allowed my six iron to come in high and land softly on the green. This thing was screaming. Luckily, it was right at my target.

Jonesy and I heard a few gasps from the onlookers behind us. For all they knew, I had almost skulled it due to the pressure. I leaned forward in my follow-through and bent my knees, pleading for the ball to land as softly as possible.

I knew I had enough to carry the bunker, and it hit the middle of the green, one-hopping over the putting surface into the rough. Honestly, this was the best-case scenario I was going to get out of the situation that I had found myself in.

Jonesy grabbed my club, filthy from the Earth. He shot me a look like what we just did was acceptable. I could have been pissed. I could have thrown a club. It was probably how I would have handled that in the past. Now, I was just happy to have a chance.

I started walking up the eighteenth hole and swore I heard my dad's cackle in the distance.

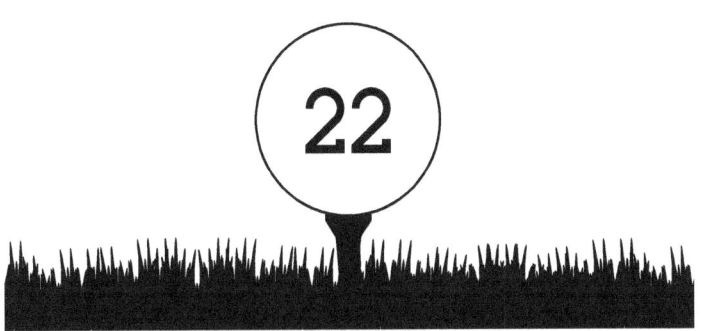

"**Y**ou are always going to be a fucking failure." The slurred words came out of Jackie's mouth right in my direction. He was angry and piss drunk. He was also frustrated trying to light his cigarette, only to realize it was backwards in his mouth and he was lighting the butt end. He threw the lighter in disgust and kept driving the car as well as he could in our lane.

His words stung, even though it was ironic that a man this intoxicated was this mad at his fourteen-year-old son for lack of success in a game.

"You're a fucking embarrassment," he continued. The vitriol in his voice grew stronger and darker. "Every fucking time you come down to the end, you piss it away. How the fuck are you going to get noticed coming in fourth or fifth? You fucking choke and shit the bed every fucking time and you cost me money. You're just a pathetic fucking excuse for a golfer."

This happened more and more as I failed on the bigger stage of junior tournaments. It made competing not fun. I began to expect every car ride to go like this. Jackie never hit me, but his words cut through my teenage soul like I had been struck directly in the face with a tire iron.

"100 yards away on eighteen and you double the hole!" He

got animated and his voice rose an octave. "They told me you would choke, and I bet a few hundred that you would be just fine. So now I have a loser fucking son and I'm out money. Do you know how that makes me feel?"

I stopped responding to these rants and kind of just allowed them to happen. There was nothing I could do anyway, and this one started to rise to a level of frustration that I hadn't heard in his voice. Part of me wanted our car to drift into oncoming traffic so I wouldn't have to hear any more of it. It was devastating to have these feelings at my age.

When we got home, Jackie fell out of the driver's seat. He was legless drunk, and I had to help him up the front steps to the couch where he lay face down and didn't move. He was out the second he hit the cushions.

I took off his shoes and brought him a blanket. Dinner hadn't even been served yet, so I went into the kitchen to see what we had to eat. There was emptiness staring at me as I opened the fridge. The only thing that was in the freezer was a bottle of Jack Daniels that Jackie must have been saving for a rainy day. Or just a day to be honest.

I looked at that bottle and pulled it out of the freezer. The black label on the bottle was cool. The brown liquor didn't look any different than a glass of Coke. I had never even taken a sip of booze despite constantly being around it. I didn't like the person it turned Jackie into but maybe I wouldn't be like that.

I took off the cap and smelled what was inside. My head reared back from the stench. It was strong and smelled like gasoline to my fourteen-year-old nostrils. Without much of a thought, I set the bottle to my lips and took a swig.

It was the first drink of my life and a long way off from the last.

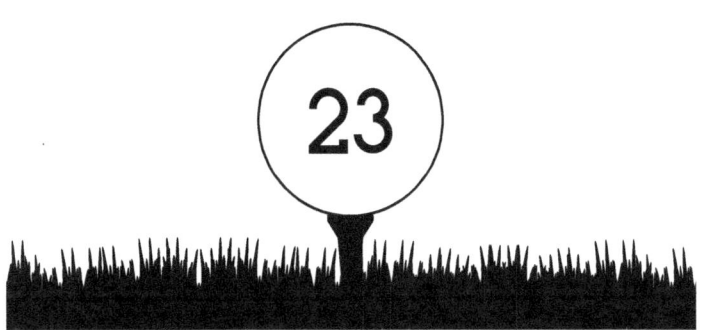

The alcohol did one of two things for me on the golf course. First, it shut down the noise that was constantly in my head. I didn't know it, but the development of my anxiety was coming on strong, especially on the golf course. Nobody teaches you that there is an active voice in your head going off twenty-four hours a day. Most of the time, it's negative. Maybe it's because no adult really knows how to deal with it either.

The second thing booze did for my young brain was give me confidence. The issues I was having closing out tournaments when I first started on the junior circuit didn't have nearly the same effect on me once I started drinking. By the time I was a junior in high school, I was back on some podiums. I wasn't winning a ton, but I wasn't completely collapsing at the end of the tournaments like I was before.

Jackie and I had better car rides. The only thing that he didn't realize, or maybe he did and was too naive to even begin to know how to handle it, was that we were both half in the bag on the drive home.

To give myself the little extra boost of mojo on the course, I would duck behind a tree and slip a sip of my drink spiked with booze. I realized I couldn't spike it too much and make it obvious that a high school kid was drinking on the course during these bigger tournaments. Nonetheless, I got pretty good at living this double life. I was a good kid on the outside, but my life was eroding slowly on the inside. At least I was making my old man a little happier with my performance.

I was running up against some of the best players in our area and at least holding my own. The competition level was certainly on the rise, and there were days I felt like I could play with anyone. Other days, I still felt like a complete failure. The inconsistencies were still there in my game. But I had enough promise to think that I could actually figure this out. If not, I would just have a drink to not give a shit either way.

I was gaining a reputation outside the golf course as a kid who liked to push the limit at parties. I was always down to get fucked up, even if I knew how unhappy it was making me the next day. There was nothing "a hair of the dog" and a chuckle out of people I barely knew that could keep me going back like the jester in the town square.

Walking up the eighteenth at Crestview, I was taking it all in. I thought a lot about that kid who was lost in life, unsure of himself in those moments, and grasping for stability and ways to manage his emotions in a healthy way.

I looked at Jonesy and realized that he was the model I should have been going after all along. The way he approached life, even when we were kids, would have set me up for way more success. But we all must walk our own path. He was a few paces ahead of me, and I didn't want to break the tension with any kind of quip or positive speech. The time for that was gone. He was feeling the pressure of what we were trying to accomplish just as much as I was.

I was living in my head and wondering what he was feeling all at the same time. His health was closer to 100 percent, but some of the muscle mass he had before never fully came back.

He and I had been through the wringer. I wish I had the

heart to tell him what I was doing to myself when we were in high school, and get the help I needed. He was on his way to Bentley and a business degree. Golf was something he was going to pursue for fun and business, and to make connections to help him in his life. If I had hitched my wagon to following in his footsteps, maybe some of that inner fortitude that he used to get through that hell just a year ago would have rubbed off on me sooner.

With each step. we were getting closer to the finality of this moment. How it would shake out, neither of us knew. I was deep in my head and remembered some of the early days of pushing Jonesy around in a wheelchair on our walks. Reggie, Jonesy, and I were just three guys in a house full of women. I'd like to think he appreciated my presence as much as I appreciated being part of his family for a little while. Jonesy and Bri were really my only family. I could feel the emotions flooding my body.

"Keep it together fuck face," I whispered to myself.

Jonesy snapped his head back as he must have sensed that I said something under my breath. I kept my head down, refraining from any eye contact with my best friend.

We started to approach the green, and I noticed that Bri and the girls were standing on the right side. I made them out first, and Jonesy lifted his head and gave them a wave shortly after. They enthusiastically returned the favor.

The smile that beamed on Jonesy's face was something that I wouldn't forget. Just a year ago, he was nearly dead. And now he was here, helping to orchestrate a round of golf for the ages. His kids were here to see him and support him, and his wife was his biggest fan.

Life was good for Jonesy. Maybe I wasn't supposed to meet him where he was all those years ago when we were just kids in a picture. Maybe whoever is calling the shots in life brings you back to exactly where you need to be in their own time. Thoughts like these always seemed to swirl to my mind in the last year. Being sober and feeling things could be overwhelming at times. But it was beautiful.

"Go see the girls, bud," I said to Jonesy and waved to the women of the Jonesy clan. "Just leave me the sixty and I'll see you over there."

Jonesy pulled the wedge out from the bag and wielded it like a knight handing over his weapon. He kept his gaze towards the girls who made up his whole life. I could tell his smile grew inexplicably wider as he walked away from me because his ears raised and his hat moved up a fraction of an inch. I was happy for my friend. I truly was. To be truly happy for another was something that my world needed more of. I surveyed the green as I walked along the edge and towards my ball.

The crowd was giving me a warm welcome and shouts of encouragement. I didn't know a soul. But, once again, I sensed a familiar set of eyes watching me.

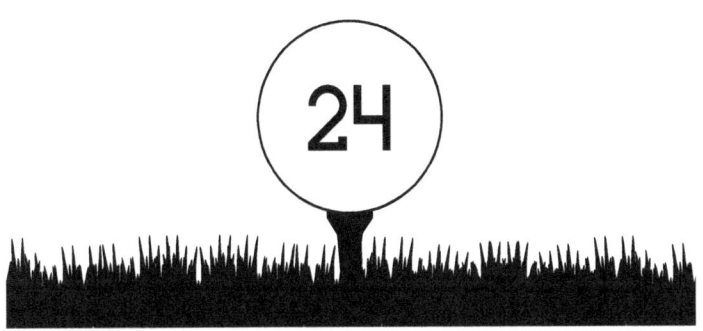

"I guess you want to know why I'm helping you out for nothing," Tom said, rocking in his chair.

He and I had grown pretty close during the last four months of this training. When he agreed to guide me in my quest for U.S. Open qualifying, we got down to business. His lessons were hard. We pushed and pushed and pushed. The stress sometimes got to me, but we always talked about keeping a simple life and sticking to a routine on the course.

I knew he was trying to make it register that I needed to do it in my life as well.

"I've thought about it a time or two," I admitted. I stopped hitting balls and leaned my weight on my club to leverage myself as I waited for his answer.

He stopped rocking but didn't stand up. He leaned forward and put his elbows on his knees. In typical Tom fashion, he didn't make full eye contact with me. This again was a listening portion of our conversation.

He told me that he had a similar upbringing to mine. He had also found solace in the game of golf and was able to escape it. His situation wasn't nearly as difficult as mine, but booze and golf hang a large shadow over his family life.

That continued later in life when he had a family of his

own. He stayed away from the life of alcohol while he raised his family. But demons sometimes skip a generation. I didn't know Tom's son. I didn't know his story. But as he told me, it sounded awfully reminiscent of my life in Florida.

When Tom saw me come back to Clark's a year ago, he noticed that I was trying. He admired it from afar in the beginning, watching someone who struggled with drugs and alcohol work his way back into a life without much guidance from anyone else. He knew my story. My hometown is not the biggest of places. He had heard about me flaming out on the mini tour and knew that I had sunk myself into my failures down in Florida.

"You gave me hope that someday my boy could come back," Tom said. He told me that he and his son had been working on things and getting his son the help that he needed. Tom wasn't an emotional man, but I could tell the weight of helplessness for his son was grinding him down. It's probably why he spent all his time giving lessons, helping others, and giving back in some kind of way.

At that moment, my respect level for Tom reached new heights (despite it already being pretty high.) For a man of his generation to be vulnerable with another human being was rare. As men, we are taught not to have emotions and keep soldiering on. As people, it's the one thing that will strip you of your ability to solve interpersonal conflicts and move towards solutions. Being alone is something that Tom was for a long time. I knew what he was feeling because I, too, felt alone. Our time allowed him to think a little differently and see his problem from a different perspective. In that, we shared something pretty special.

I wasn't sure what to say.

"What you have done for me can't be put into words, sir," I took off my cap and reached out my hand.

He grabbed it firmly and finally made eye contact.

"I need you to do something, kid," Tom said.

"Anything," I said. I felt like I owed him my life in many ways.

"Now it's your turn to bury the hatchet with your old man," he said. "It's the last lesson you'll ever need from me."

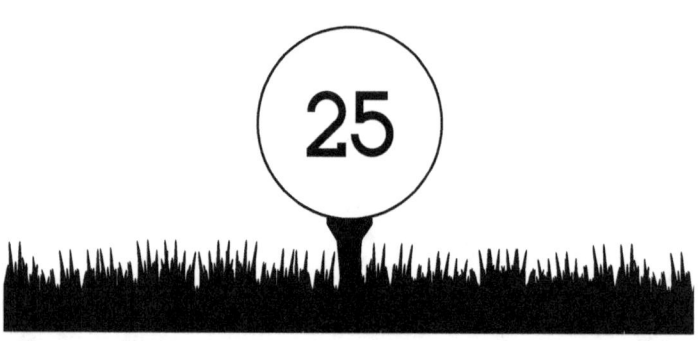

25

Stepping back into Ridgeway was like going back in time. The smells were familiar, even though I hadn't been there in more than two decades. I didn't feel like an adult. I felt like I was that kid again, shuffling up the stairs after a long day of work on my game, wondering when I would be able to get my dad out of the bar.

The plaques with the names of the past club champions lined the hallway up the stairs. I stopped and let my eyes linger on the one for the juniors. Jake Steadman, six years running. I felt like it wasn't even me who did that. Like it was another person who was part of me, but not anymore. I continued up the stairs towards the main dining room. Sweat was starting to form on my brow. A tightness around my neck and shoulders developed quickly. To get to the back deck, where I was certain my old man would be, I had to pass right through the bar.

It was quiet. Most Mondays at the club were. The week-enders were all back to their lives with work and family and responsibilities. The bar wasn't buzzing. Debauchery wasn't happening. Jackie's sermons certainly weren't taking place.

I could see a figure in a familiar seat through the window, and a pain hit me in the gut. The voice in my head was telling me to go the other way. He hadn't seen me yet.

"Look what the cat dragged in," called a voice from behind the bar.

I hadn't even noticed Tony, the longtime bartender at Ridgeway, standing there cleaning glasses. That's how focused I was on my old man. He was still transfixed by the green on the eighteenth hole, unaware that I was less than twenty feet from him for the first time in a very long time.

"Tony, it's great to see you, man. Been a long time," I extended my hand and did my best to put on a face. Tony was the guy who overserved my dad daily for the last forty-something years. He was just doing his job. But in some ways, I wondered if he knew the carnage he created with the one-more mentality that he enabled from a lot of people at Ridgeway. Got to pay the bills, I guess.

"You know, kid. Same old shit, different day," Tony said. "Your old man is out back in his usual spot. Can I get you anything?"

"Nah, I'm good. But thank you," I replied.

"Always, Mr. Polite, Jakey. It's been a long fucking time my friend. Your old man talks about you all the time," he said.

This surprised me. There were no tall tales to tell about me in the last decade. I wondered what kind of stories he could be telling about me, or if Tony was just saying it to be nice.

"How's he doing?" I asked Tony. At this point, I was just making small talk, but I could also use whatever intel I could get before I actually approached my father.

"The old man?" Tony said. "He's the same as he's ever been. He's slowed down a ton, but he hasn't missed a day here at the club in years. He ain't playing much golf anymore, that's for sure. But that's his perch out there. I fuck with him and tell him that he's turning into an owl. I know when he needs another one when he turns his head towards the bar."

That's Tony for you. Unaware of the gasoline he was throwing on Jackie all these years. He sure as hell didn't have to deal with the consequences. As long as the guys tipped well and took care of him, it didn't matter.

"Thanks, Tony. And it was good to see you. Mind if I grab a water while you're at it?" I asked.

Tony poured the water halfway and scooped ice into the rest of the glass before topping it off. My mouth was starting to go dry as the moment of truth started to approach. I threw a few bucks down on the bar and headed out towards the deck.

It was a beautiful day, and there was a group coming up on the eighteenth. It was probably some old retirees who spent all their time at the club, just like Jackie. The old man was hunched over with his arms leaning on the rail. He was frailer than I remember, not nearly the hulking figure that I recall when I was a kid. The cigar smoke bellowed into the air, and I noticed his thick head of hair wasn't as plush as it used to be. Age was hitting Jackie hard. It was like looking at a different human being.

"I heard you've been back in town for a while," Jackie said. He had this uncanny ability, like Tom did, to speak to you or know of your presence even if you hadn't officially made eye contact yet. The conversation that was fifteen years in the making was commencing.

"Yes, sir. I came back when Jonesy got sick and decided to stay. He and Bri needed help..."

He picked up his nearly empty glass. Brown liquor. Who knew where this conversation was going to go?

"So, I've been staying there until I figure out next steps," I finished my thought.

"Mmmmm," Jackie kind of grunted. "You didn't think to come by and see your old man or visit your old friends here at the club?" Jackie's tone was dark. It was like those long car rides home. I knew this would probably be a short conversation. The best thing to do was to hit it head-on.

"I needed time for myself. I'm here now, though," I said. I was proud of how firm I was in my answer. This was hard. But deep breathing and falling back on all the things I've learned in the past year were going to get me through this.

"I heard you're playing again. Heard that Tom Clark was giving you lessons. Never liked that know-it-all," he said.

Jackie was one to talk.

"Yes sir. I'm playing well and going to try for local qualifying for the U.S. Open next month," I said.

"Heard that too," he said.

There was a long pause next. I moved up to the railing and grabbed some space next to him. We both watched the golfers putting out on eighteen. One of the guys lipped out for his par and let out a curse word like any good native New Englander. The group finished out the hole and removed their hats before shaking hands.

Golf has so many unwritten rules in how to conduct yourself on the golf course: don't throw clubs, don't scuff up the greens, be quiet when your playing partners are hitting. Respect. Honesty. Truth. All of it. The handshake was one of my favorites. No matter what happened out there for eighteen holes, you needed to look your opponent in the eye and shake their hand.

The way this back-and-forth was going, there was not going to be any kumbaya moment. I wasn't even sure what I wanted to get out of this now that I think about it. Honestly, it was more of just my willingness to come back to Ridgeway and extend the first olive branch.

"You want a drink?" Jackie said. His voice wasn't as powerful as it used to be. I could tell where he was headed after a few more rounds.

"I'm good, pop. I quit a year ago. Been clean for thirteen months," I said.

"Hmmmm," Jackie shrugged it off and took a long pause. "Well, I'll see you around, kid. Got to take a piss."

Just like that, he got up from the seat and walked into the restaurant. His first stop wasn't to the bathroom; it was straight to Tony. I watched Tony pull a bottle from behind the bar and realized that was my cue to go.

Jackie's half-lit cigar burned right there in the ashtray. I collected my pride and walked down the back steps and out of Ridgeway for maybe the last time.

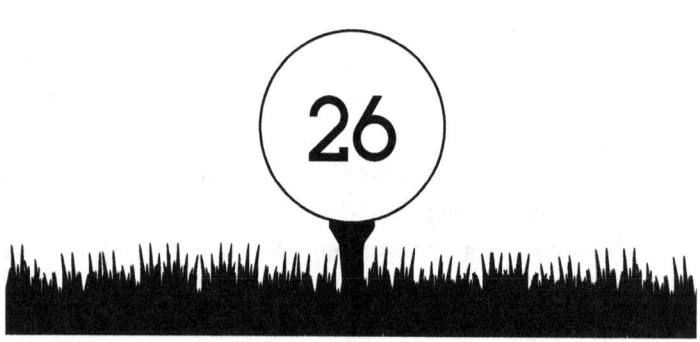

26

"What's the play here, bud?" Jonesy asked as he walked over towards me. You couldn't wipe the shit eating grin off his face if you wanted to right now. I felt proud of how far he'd come and how much having his family there meant to him.

The job was not finished, however, and Jonesy had a way of locking back in when he knew there was still something left to be done.

The pin was tucked on the front part of the green, which made my decision to play long out of the lie that I had all the easier. Looking back from this angle, there was no way in hell I was going to be able to get enough loft on the ball to stop it. The front bunker would have been hell to get up and down from, looking from this side. All things considered, I was happy with where I was.

The green sloped severely from front to back. I only had one option. I needed to land this ball on the fringe and let it trickle down towards the hole. A bump and run would pick up too much speed, and I'd have a twenty-five-footer coming back up the hill. Ideally, I'd want to get lucky and have something within a foot to knock it in and get the hell out of here with the spot secured. But with the lie, the situation, and the way this green shot straight downhill, I would take inside fifteen feet just to give myself a chance.

Jonesy and I picked our spot and the rest was up to me. I did my best to keep the crowd at my back the entire time to block out just how many people were around to watch me succeed or fail. I glanced up back at the tee box and realized I had replayed my entire life up to this moment. It couldn't have been more than twelve minutes of actual time from the moment we teed off to where I was now, but it felt like an eternity. I smiled. It felt good to do that. As I scanned around to really soak in the last memories of this, I noticed a figure standing against a tree in the distance.

It was Tom.

I had no idea he was even here. It was unexpected, and I could feel a lump in my throat. The first thing that stood out to me was his positioning. He wasn't front and center like Jackie. His voice couldn't be heard by me. He wasn't even saying anything or standing with anyone. Tom was the steady voice that I needed in my life, and I gave him a nod without losing too much of my concentration.

I took the sixty-degree and set it behind the ball. I knew I needed to open the face as much as I could to get the ball to pop up and land soft where it needed to. I picked the club up and came in as steep as I possibly could to generate spin. The ball popped up straight into the air, and I got a little too much on it. The ball missed my mark by half a foot and started darting towards the hole.

I could do nothing but watch as gravity decided where the ball wanted to come to rest.

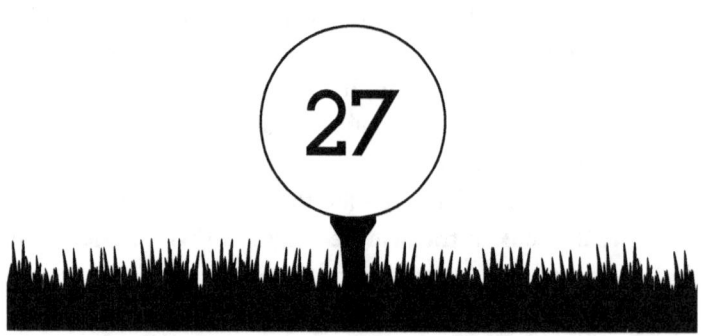

I sat in the car in front of Jonesy's for a few minutes after my unsuccessful meeting with my old man at the club. This was one of those sits in the car where you do nothing, say nothing, and just be.

What happened at the club hurt more than I wanted to let on. I felt betrayed. I shouldn't have expected some warm embrace or anything other than what happened. It was just the coldness of it all. My thoughts started coming at me quickly. I wondered if I should have tried in the last year to meet him sooner than I did. Maybe. Probably. Shoulda, coulda, woulda.

Right now, was the exact moment I'd reach for a substance, to just put my mind at ease and not feel a fucking thing. This new version of me was different, and sometimes sitting in discomfort was the only thing that could get me out of it.

Jonesy and Bri were home with the kids and probably wondered what I was doing in the driveway for the last ten minutes. I turned off the engine and walked into the house.

"How did it go?" Jonesy asked after a few quiet moments in the kitchen. Bri and Jonesy were both sitting at the kitchen table, looking like concerned parents. They knew I was going to take on this feat today and waited all day for me to get home to hear how it went. I think they were just happy I wasn't bellied up at the bar somewhere getting the edge off.

"It went…" My voice began to trail off. My lip quivered. Bri and Jonesy looked at each other, sensing my world caving in.

"I just don't know what to do about it anymore," and all of a sudden, it all came flooding out. "I shouldn't have been surprised or even hoping that he would be a changed person. There's been no reason for him to make a change. I was just hoping that maybe seeing me turn my life around, or at least hearing that I was turning my life around, would make him proud. But it made him nothing. It made him not seem to give a fuck about me or my life or my existence. I could have been a complete stranger for that matter or just someone taking his fucking drink order." Bri and Jonesy said nothing. They let me keep going.

"All my life I've wanted something from that man. And to get nothing is something that is going to haunt me the rest of my life. The times I was basically dying down in Florida, and he did nothing to acknowledge it. I needed a fucking father in my life. I got the one I got. And that's something I'll have to live with. There were times a year ago when I actively thought about not being around anymore."

Jonesy squirmed a bit in his chair. I hadn't told a soul about what I was planning on doing.

"I just," tears had been pouring without me even realizing it. The emotions that were built up and stuffed away under the guise of drugs and alcohol had burst to the surface like a volcano erupting.

"I just want to know why I'm not enough. Why am I not enough?"

I put my head down, and both Bri and Jonesy came and embraced me. Just a few years ago, Bri wouldn't even let Jonesy mention me as a guest at their wedding. Now here I was in their kitchen as a member of a family, the first one I had ever felt a part of. The moment was cathartic and needed. It felt like it was one of the last stages of my recovery back

to life and my chance to finally let go.
Or at least I thought so.

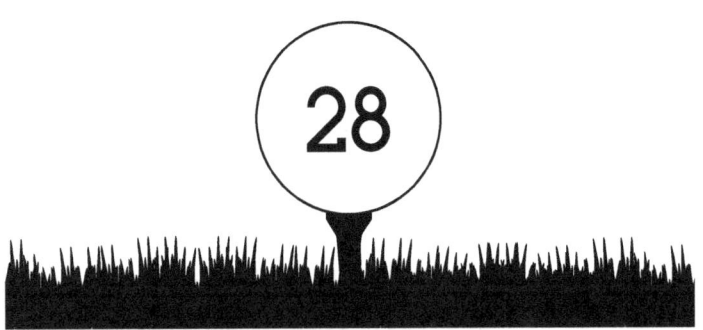

Later that night, I took Reggie on a long walk without my phone and Jonesy. I needed to be alone. Well, not completely. This dog was one of the true blessings of my life last year, and he was great company. He didn't talk back. He just needed a little bit of attention. The walks also got my body moving forward and out of my head for a little bit.

I needed no distraction, so I left my phone in the kitchen.

It was a crisp April night in New England. The kind where you could tell that warmer days were coming, but winter was still trying to hang on. I could still faintly see my breath in the night air.

A lot was going through my mind: lots of anger, lots of disappointment, some relief. Deep down, I had been hanging on to this fairy tale ending for mine and Jackie's story. It wasn't something I talked about. It was always part of me since I was a little kid. It was why I tried so hard to be noticed when I was just a kid at Ridgeway. It was probably why I started drinking and smoking and taking drugs. I wanted someone to say to me that this was not alright. A little discipline would have gone a long way. I finished my loop with Reggie and decided to move back towards the house. The back deck lights were on, and I could see Jonesy waiting outside.

He wasn't usually out there. Reggie ran ahead of me off leash towards the house and let out a bark for Jonesy.

When I got close, he had a very concerned look in his eyes.

"Hey, bud, Mike called," he said. "Something happened to your dad. He's in the hospital. Mike has all the details, and he's been blowing up your phone."

A sinking feeling bloomed in the pit of my stomach. Deep down, I hoped that the last time I spoke to my dad would be on the back patio of the club.

I got to my phone and saw how many texts and missed calls I had from Mike. He must have been my old man's emergency contact. He seemed to have his pulse on everything, even from Florida.

Mike picked up on the first ring.

"Kid, where have you been?" he said.

"Sorry, Mike. I was out on a walk with the dog and needed to be away from everything. I saw my pops today at the club, and it didn't go well," I said.

"I heard. Well, your old man really tied one on when you left. Tony told me it was the worst he had seen him in years," Mike said. "Tony tried to get him to not drive home, but you know Jackie. He's as stubborn as a fucking mule. He almost got back home but crashed his car head-on into a telephone pole. The car is totaled and he's..."

I waited for Mike to tell me he was dead.

"...pretty banged up and down at South Shore Hospital. He should make a full recovery, but he was asking about you before they put him under to work on his injuries. He cracked a few ribs and broke his shoulder. He's also cut up pretty bad."

"Jesus, fucking Christ," was all I could say.

"Listen, kid," Mike said. "I never got involved with what was between you and your old man. I know he's no fucking saint. He had it pretty hard after your mother passed away. He was never one for feelings after that, even though deep down, I know he had them. Your old man is a good person.

He's just got a problem. And he didn't know how to be your dad when your shit started heading south."

I shuddered to think what Mike found in my apartment the morning I had to leave in a hurry to get home to see Jonesy a year ago.

"It was your old man who gave me money to make sure you had a place to stay. He would send me your rent every month, and all that cash I was able to hand you was the money I saved when you were actually able to pay me on time."

I felt like a piece of shit. A drink sounded good right about now.

"He asked about you a lot. Sure, he was half in the bag most of the time when he asked, but you were still on his mind. I know you don't see it this way, probably from years of feeling you were being wronged, but he did care for you. It was sloppy the way he tried to love you, but it was really the only way he knew how and all he could give."

Mike sounded like a man who knew something about apologies and acceptance.

"I'm not telling you what to do, but when you go up there, just remember that. At the end of the day, family is all we've got. The family we create along the way is amazing, too. But that's your old man, and you are his only thing he might have left for the time he's still got with us. Just try to remember that kid, when you go see him."

I let that land a bit and said nothing for a moment.

"Thanks, Mike. You're a good friend to him...and to me."

"Anytime, kid," he said in his matter-of-fact way. "I'll always be here, just let me know what you need me to do."

I hung up the phone and turned towards the house. Jonesy was already outside with my coat and his keys. We were off to the hospital.

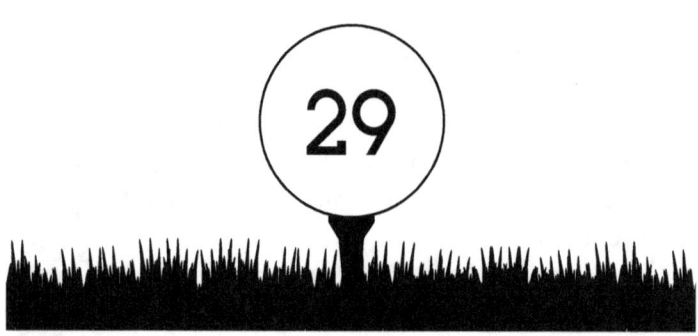

Watching that ball roll down towards the hole was like watching something happen in slow motion. I knew I had missed my mark, and I was just hoping that I would have something makeable on the other end. The crowd willed the ball to stop. The nervous energy emanating from those around the green was palpable.

I knew Tom hadn't moved an inch from where he stood in the sea of madness. Neither did I.

The roller coaster ride started right on track, but the slope of the green carried the ball past the right side of the cup. It had a good amount of pace on it, but I knew I'd hold the green. It was a few centimeters from being an absolutely perfect shot. Such is life in the game of golf.

The ball nestled some twelve feet away from the hole. That is what I would have left to finalize the last spot and a chance at redemption for the life I had lived up to this point.

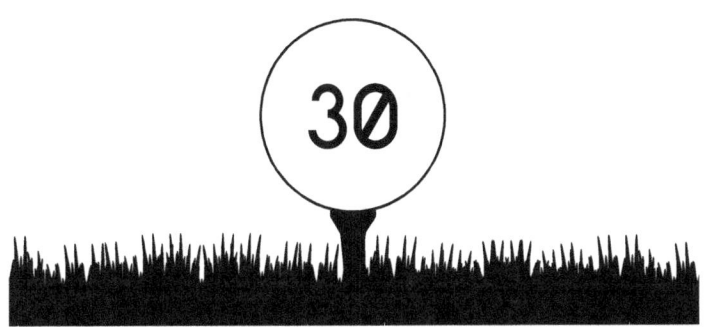

Walking into that hospital felt like déjà vu. The feeling of the unknown, of what I was walking into, felt just like the day I came back home to find Jonesy nearly lifeless in a hospital bed.

I remember thinking it should be me when I looked at Jonesy. When I saw my dad in his bed, I was determined to never have to walk into a situation like this again.

The nurse told me that he would be a little bit groggy and that they had put him under to help him sleep. He was still shitfaced when they brought him in and was coming down from his drunkenness. They pumped him full of fluids and needed to wait until he came down from the alcohol before they could give him a full dose of medication to help manage his pain.

"Your dad is a lucky guy," the nurse said. "Someone must have been up there watching over him."

Maybe so.

I entered the room, and he was still asleep. I took a seat next to the bed and waited for him to move. Looking over his body, there wasn't much of the man I remember from my childhood. The way he would hold court and stand tall when talking about himself, or me, after a few beverages at Ridgeway was something he probably couldn't even muster up the strength to do anymore. That generation had also left the club, so he was just a legend living amongst a new generation of people who didn't know much about him other than the stories they heard. It was no wonder that I found him sitting by himself in his old spot earlier that day when we had our first meeting. I bet that, alone, was killing him. Our conversation probably didn't help and drove him over the edge.

I wasn't sure what I would say to him when he did eventually wake up. How would I handle this? Should I be mad and move on with my life? Or would it make sense to see what could happen and make amends, even if it was just temporarily, until he could get back on his feet?

The Red Sox game was on the television in the room, and I sat there and waited until I nodded off. The heaviness of the day had been getting to me, too. I don't know how long I was out, but I heard Jackie start to move in his bed. I came to my senses. He was staring straight up at the ceiling, probably confused as to where he was. He couldn't move his body all that much because of the broken ribs and the whiplash from the accident.

He took a deep inhale, and I could hear how it pained him.

"Pop," I said. It seemed to startle him a bit.

"Kid? That you?" he said, feeling around with his right hand. He made contact with my hand, and we embraced for the first time, maybe ever. His grip was light, and there was no power behind it. He was completely vulnerable, and it was the first time I had seen him like this, with real fear in his eyes. My shoulders let go, and my guard dropped.

"Yeah, pop. It's me."

His grip tightened slightly. His breath was unsteady in and out.

"I'm sorry, kid. I'm sorry." Jackie shut his eyes and rested. A tear trickled out of his right eye. He lay there as comfortably as he could and didn't let go of my hand.

I stayed there with him through the night. It was enough

to turn the page. My anger towards my father was gone. Whatever path we took after that, the apology was all I needed to move forward.

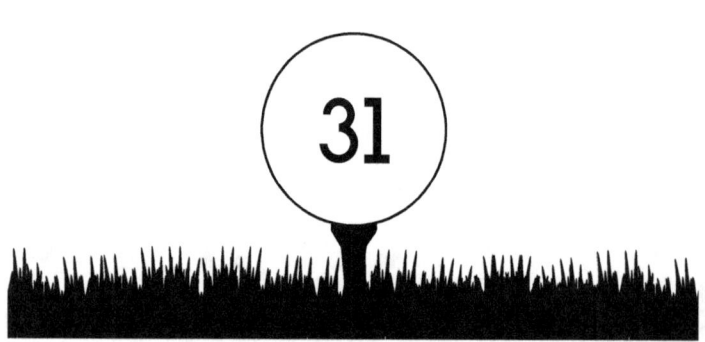

31

There was a smattering of applause when the ball came to rest. It wasn't the loudest one, and I'm not sure it was even warranted. At least I was below the hole.

I tracked my route from behind the hole and went to put a mark on my ball. I pulled out a marker from Ridgeway. Jackie asked me to use it to remember where we came from. He had been recovering nicely over the last couple of weeks and was able to go home. I helped him like I had helped Jonesy. It felt good for me to give back. Having that purpose and having this tournament on the calendar allowed me to lock in like I had never done before.

I put the coin down and picked up my ball. I crouched into a squat like a catcher in baseball and passed the ball behind my head. Jonesy was there reading the putt already. I always knew he had my back.

All that stood between me and a spot in the next round of U.S. Open qualifying was this twelve-foot putt. It was uphill so I knew I needed to give it some pace. There was a little bit of left to right swing in it at the end.

"Don't give up the cup," Jonesy said without missing a beat.

I agreed and studied intensely for the line to speak to me while my playing partners played their shots.

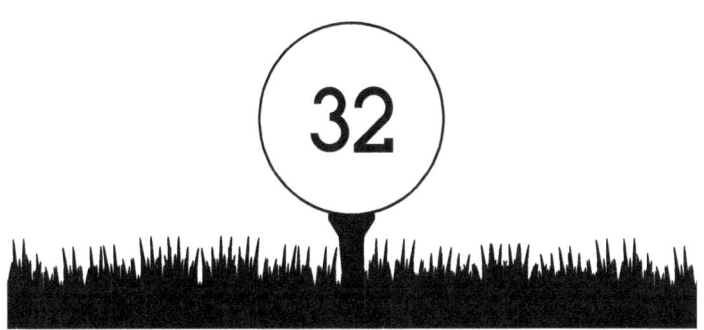

There was a voicemail on my phone for a few days that I hadn't gotten around to listening to yet. I was bellied up at a bar for what felt like a week. I had no concept of time. I'm not sure if I drank or ate food for several days. The only thing I could taste was the drip of cocaine hitting the back of my throat.

"Mr. Steadman. This is Sean down at Sean's Hunting and Fishing. Your order is ready, and you can pick it up at your convenience. Thank you and have a great day."

The voice was unfamiliar. The reason for the call was not. There was only one way that I was going to be able to escape my miserable existence, and it took me some time to figure out if this was the way. Any time I tried to not be fucked up, the voices and doubt in my head would get so loud that the only way to block it out was to keep the party going or blow my brains out.

The latter was now turning into my last and only option.

I had not heard from anyone in my life for weeks at a time. The only people I encountered were the deadbeats and burnouts I would meet in establishments like the one I was in. I was in my mid-thirties with no friends, no family, no purpose, and no discernible skills that would get me out of the predicament that I was in. To me, there was no other choice. My cry for help wouldn't be heard by anyone.

Action was the only thing that would put my mind at ease.

I picked up the gun the next morning and did my best to keep my composure.

"Have a great day, Mr. Steadman," the cashier said. "We appreciate your business." I'm sure you fucking do pal.

The plan was to grab more than enough beer, several bottles of uppers and downers, a rock of cocaine, and this pistol. One of the things would ultimately do me in. I got back to my apartment, and Mike's light was on. I didn't want to bother him. I felt bad for what he would ultimately be responsible for. But I was selfish and dammit I wanted to be. Maybe the old man would give two fucks about me now.

The first order was to swallow down a few of these pills as quickly as possible and get the party started. I cracked my first beer of this sitting, certainly not of the day, and threw some painkillers back and down my throat. The swig of my first sip went down too fast. I was in this thing to see it through.

I cut out a fat line of cocaine on a mirror and took it down like I had done so many times. My head kicked back, and a rush of adrenaline surged through my body. I got to my feet and threw some punches into the air. Jake Steadman, the showman, was here to put on his final act.

The uneasiness didn't take long to kick in. Mixing uppers and downers wasn't a new thing for me. The amount I put in my body at this one time was. I kept slugging back my drinks and turned on the game.

There were pizza boxes and shit all over the apartment. I hadn't cleaned it in God knows how long. I was fucked up. The true end was officially starting to come into play. I grabbed the gun and stared at it. There were three at this time, and my vision was becoming incredibly unsteady. I waved the gun around to see if it was me or if I had bought three guns at the store just a few hours ago.

I put the pistol to my mouth. Then under my chin. Then next to my temple. I had no idea how one would go through with killing themselves. I shoved the gun deep into my throat and gagged. My finger wasn't on the trigger yet. I was just practicing.

I turned the volume up on the TV when I finally figured out where the remote was. My phone buzzed, and I threw it as hard as I could towards the kitchen. Fuck that thing. Nobody was calling me anyways.

I placed the gun back down on the table and stared straight ahead at the TV. Emotions were swirling now. I started to say something but couldn't make it out. I'm not sure my brain was even comprehending what was happening at that moment.

I grabbed the gun one more time. This was really going to be my end. A nothing. A nobody. A never was. Jake Steadman would be in the newspaper again. This time, it would be for an obituary if anyone ever felt like filing a death certificate in the first place.

I tried to stand up but fell back down on the couch. I laughed. Hysterically. The gun fell out of my hand, and I could feel the walls caving in. It was the last thing I remembered until I woke up the next morning. The TV was loud, and I could hear a vibration coming from somewhere in the kitchen.

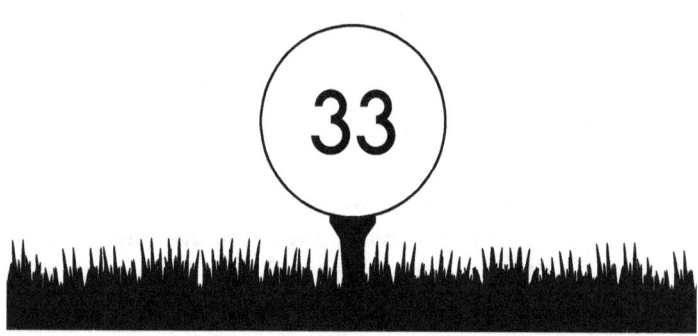

33

Bri was in my line of sight as I continued to line up my putt. She was staring nervously towards the green. The girls flanked her sides. Without her phone call that morning, I would have eventually followed through on whatever my plan was that night.

I'm so grateful she made that call.

It wasn't even about being out here living out a childhood dream. It was about being alive. It was about getting a second chance. Life is about more than one second of greatness. I now had multiple moments to be great. My definition of those moments changed over the last year. Helping a friend get to the bathroom to take a piss was a moment of greatness. Spending time with a dog who helped change my life was a moment of greatness. The act of loving, crying, laughing, and feeling emotions were great experiences to live out. Giving people hope in me and trusting that I would come through when they needed me were maybe some of the greatest moments of all.

Life isn't about the big wins. It's about the times you get a chance to go after the things you want and stay true to who you are and who you want to become. I knew what this putt was going to do. I had seen this putt before in so many hours on the practice green from when I was just a boy to when I put my head down and worked to get to this moment.

The crowd around the green was dead silent. My playing partners had finished up out of respect for the moment I was potentially about to have. I couldn't bring myself to look in Tom's direction. But I knew he was there. So was Jonesy and Bri. So was my old man, in spirit. I looked up in the sky, in the direction where he would have perched himself for the event He wasn't there, but I wasn't angry. I was hoping that I would give him a chance to host a sermon again with his friends down at the rehab clinic where he was getting his life back.

"Give it a little pace and make sure it holds the line," was my only golf thought I needed.

I lined up my putter towards my target. I had it in my sights. I took one last deep breath and pulled the putter back.

This last second of greatness was just the beginning of the rest of my life.

THE END

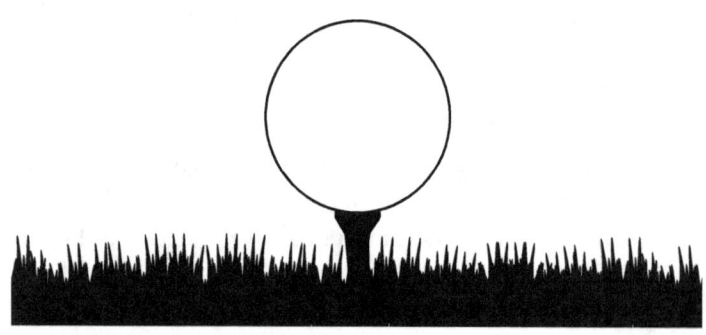

Acknowledgements

This project was a lifetime in the making and there are many people to thank for their special place in my life and in the creation of this book.

Thank you to Stacy Padula and Briley & Baxter Publications for believing in this story and the message we all hope it conveys to the people who read these pages. To Stacy, I thank you. Grabbing coffee two years ago was one of the best decisions I've ever made.

To my family for their continued support and love. You have all been there since day one and have followed me through my ups and downs. I appreciate you all and especially to my brother Jay for the cover design of Level Par.

To my dog, Reggie. It might sound funny to thank a dog. But not to me. You changed my life and any time I was hung up or questioning where to go with this story and what to do with this book we worked it out on a long, morning walk. For that, I am grateful.

To Tom Cavicchi for your golf lessons and for your inspiration to write this story. I'm still not sure I'll ever get rid of some of my bad golf habits, but you are helping me out in more ways than you know. Honored to work with you in this lifelong pursuit of playing better golf.

To Brian Fabry, Danny Ventura and Hank Hryniewicz for giving me a shot at starting my writing career at the Boston Herald. I had zero writing experience and had nothing to show when I came in for that first interview. But you needed a guy to answer phones, and you took a chance on me. Hank, you told me to never stop bringing you stories. I hope this one is the "best evah!"

To my professors at Emerson College for teaching me how to be a better storyteller and to think critically. Thank you for all that you have done.

To Kristy Dupuis for being my first-ever editor for Level Par. Your students are very lucky to have you as their teacher and I'm lucky to call you a friend.

To Arnout Schepers for always asking me when I was going to start writing the book. I didn't always have the answer you wanted, but I'm not sure this project gets done without that thoughtful Dutch needling to think bigger. Thank you, my friend.

To Mike and PJ. I hope I'm making you boys proud. Cheers to the studs.

Lastly, I want to thank you, the reader. Thank you for reading my words. You picked up this book for whatever reason. Maybe I know you personally. Maybe you are family. Maybe you are just one of the crazy ones who love golf and wanted to read a story about this beautiful game. Whatever your reason, I hope this story helps you in some way. I hope you realize, like I am continuing to try to do so, that the journey is always more important than the result. Finding out who you are and what you are made of will always beat the score on the card.

www.ingramcontent.com/pod-product-compliance
Lightning Source LLC
Chambersburg PA
CBHW061702120626
46550CB00003B/1060